Urinary Tract Infections: Diagnostic and Management Issues

Editor

KALPANA GUPTA

INFECTIOUS DISEASE CLINICS OF NORTH AMERICA

www.id.theclinics.com

Consulting Editor
HELEN W. BOUCHER

March 2014 • Volume 28 • Number 1

ELSEVIER

1600 John F. Kennedy Boulevard • Suite 1800 • Philadelphia, Pennsylvania, 19103-2899.
http://www.theclinics.com

INFECTIOUS DISEASE CLINICS OF NORTH AMERICA Volume 28, Number 1
March 2014 ISSN 0891–5520, ISBN-13: 978-0-323-28708-1

Editor: Jessica McCool
Developmental Editor: Donald Mumford

Infectious Disease Clinics of North America (ISSN 0891–5520) is published in March, June, September, and December by Elsevier Inc., 360 Park Avenue South, New York, NY 10010-1710. Periodicals postage paid at New York, NY and additional mailing offices. Subscription prices are $295.00 per year for US individuals, $510.00 per year for US institutions, $145.00 per year for US students, $350.00 per year for Canadian individuals, $638.00 per year for Canadian institutions, $420.00 per year for international individuals, $638.00 per year for international institutions, and $200.00 per year for Canadian and international students. To receive student rate, orders must be accompanied by name of affiliated institution, date of term, and the *signature* of program/residency coordinator on institution letterhead. Orders will be billed at individual rate until proof of status is received. Foreign air speed delivery is included in all *Clinics* subscription prices. All prices are subject to change without notice. **POSTMASTER**: Send address changes to *Infectious Disease Clinics of North America*, Elsevier Health Sciences Division, Subcription Customer Service, 3251 Riverport Lane, Maryland Heights, MO 63043. **Customer Service: 1-800-654-2452 (US). From outside of the US and Canada, call 1-314-447-8871. Fax: 1-314-447-8029. E-mail: JournalsCustomerService-usa@elsevier.com (print support) or JournalsOnlineSupport-usa@elsevier.com (online support).**

Infectious Disease Clinics of North America is also published in Spanish by Editorial Inter-Médica, Junin 917, 1ᵉʳ A 1113, Buenos Aires, Argentina.

Reprints. For copies of 100 or more, of articles in this publication, please contact the Commercial Reprints Department, Elsevier Inc., 360 Park Avenue South, New York, New York 10010-1710. Tel. 212-633-3874, Fax: 212-633-3820, E-mail: reprints@elsevier.com.

Infectious Disease Clinics of North America is covered in *MEDLINE/PubMed (Index Medicus), Current Contents/Clinical Medicine, Science Citation Alert, SCISEARCH,* and *Research Alert.*

Printed and bound by CPI Group (UK) Ltd, Croydon, CR0 4YY

Contributors

CONSULTING EDITOR

HELEN W. BOUCHER, MD, FIDSA, FACP
Director, Infectious Diseases Fellowship Program; Associate Professor of Medicine, Division of Geographic Medicine and Infectious Diseases, Tufts Medical Center, Boston, Massachusetts

EDITOR

KALPANA GUPTA, MD, MPH
Chief, Infectious Diseases, VA Boston HCS, West Roxbury; Associate Professor, Infectious Diseases, Boston University School of Medicine, Boston, Massachusetts

AUTHORS

MARIËLLE A.J. BEEREPOOT, MD, PhD
Division of Infectious Diseases, Department of Internal Medicine, Academic Medical Center, Amsterdam, The Netherlands

NAHID BHADELIA, MD, MA
Associate Director of Hospital Epidemiology, Assistant Professor, Section of Infectious Diseases, Boston Medical Center, Boston University School of Medicine, Boston, Massachusetts

CAROL E. CHENOWETH, MD
Division of Infectious Diseases, Department of Internal Medicine, University of Michigan Health System, Ann Arbor, Michigan

ELODI J. DIELUBANZA, MD
Department of Urology, Feinberg School of Medicine, Northwestern University, Chicago, Illinois

BETSY FOXMAN, PhD
Hunein F. and Hilda Maassab Professor of Epidemiology, Director, Center for Molecular and Clinical Epidemiology of Infectious Diseases, University of Michigan School of Public Health, Ann Arbor, Michigan

SUZANNE E. GEERLINGS, MD, PhD
Division of Infectious Diseases, Department of Internal Medicine, Academic Medical Center, Amsterdam, The Netherlands

CAROLYN V. GOULD, MD, MSCR
Centers for Disease Control and Prevention, Atlanta, Georgia

LARISSA GRIGORYAN, MD, PhD
Department of Family and Community Medicine, Baylor College of Medicine, Houston, Texas

KALPANA GUPTA, MD, MPH
Chief, Infectious Diseases, VA Boston HCS, West Roxbury; Associate Professor, Infectious Diseases, Boston University School of Medicine, Boston, Massachusetts

MANISHA JUTHANI-MEHTA, MD
Associate Professor of Medicine, Section of Infectious Diseases, Department of Internal Medicine, Yale University School of Medicine, New Haven, Connecticut

CAROL A. KAUFFMAN, MD
Chief, Infectious Diseases Section, Veterans Affairs Ann Arbor Healthcare System; Professor of Internal Medicine, University of Michigan Medical School, Ann Arbor, Michigan

DANIEL J. MAZUR, MD
Department of Urology, Feinberg School of Medicine, Northwestern University, Chicago, Illinois

GREGORY J. MORAN, MD, FACEP, FAAEM, FIDSA
Clinical Professor of Medicine, Department of Emergency Medicine and Division of Infectious Diseases, Olive View-UCLA Medical Center, Geffen School of Medicine at UCLA, Los Angeles, California

LINDSAY E. NICOLLE, MD, FRCPC
Professor of Internal Medicine, Medical Microbiology, University of Manitoba, Winnipeg, Manitoba, Canada

JAN M. PRINS, MD, PhD
Division of Infectious Diseases, Department of Internal Medicine, Academic Medical Center, Amsterdam, The Netherlands

THERESA ANNE ROWE, DO
Infectious Disease Fellow, Yale University School of Medicine, New Haven, Connecticut

SANJAY SAINT, MD, MPH
Division of General Medicine, Department of Internal Medicine, University of Michigan Health System and the Veterans Affairs Ann Arbor Healthcare System, Ann Arbor, Michigan

ANTHONY J. SCHAEFFER, MD
Chair, Department of Urology, Feinberg School of Medicine, Northwestern University, Chicago, Illinois

ANN E. STAPLETON, MD, FACP
Professor, Division of Allergy and Infectious Diseases, Department of Medicine; Medical Director, Clinical Research Center, Institute of Translational Health Sciences, University of Washington, Seattle, Washington

SUKHJIT S. TAKHAR, MD
Instructor of Medicine (Emergency Medicine), Department of Emergency Medicine, Brigham and Women's Hospital, Harvard Medical School, Boston, Massachusetts

BARBARA W. TRAUTNER, MD, PhD
Investigator, Center for Innovations in Quality, Effectiveness and Safety (IQuESt), Michael E. DeBakey Veterans Affairs Medical Center; Department of Medicine, Section of Infectious Diseases, Baylor College of Medicine, Houston, Texas

Contents

> Urinary tract infection (UTI) is one of the most common bacterial infections, accounting for 0.9% of all ambulatory visits in the United States. This review defines the major UTI syndromes, their occurrence and recurrence, bacteriology, risk factors, and disease burden.

> Asymptomatic bacteriuria (ASB) is a condition in which bacteria are present in a noncontaminated urine sample collected from a patient without signs or symptoms related to the urinary tract. ASB must be distinguished from symptomatic urinary tract infection (UTI) by the absence of signs and symptoms compatible with UTI or by clinical determination that a nonurinary cause accounts for the patient's symptoms. The overall purpose of this review is to promote an awareness of ASB as a distinct condition from UTI and to empower clinicians to withhold antibiotics in situations in which antimicrobial treatment of bacteriuria is not indicated.

> Emergency physicians encounter urinary tract infections (UTIs) in a wide spectrum of disease severity and patient populations. The challenges of managing UTIs in an emergency department include limited history, lack of follow-up, and lack of culture and susceptibility results. Most patients do not require an extensive diagnostic evaluation and can be safely managed as outpatients with oral antibiotics. The diagnostic approach to and treatment of adults presenting to emergency departments with UTIs are reviewed.

> Antibiotic resistance worsens clinical outcomes and, in some cases, significantly impacts the clinical management of urinary tract infections in the outpatient setting. This article presents the prevalence and mechanism of relevant antimicrobial resistance patterns encountered among uropathogens, and discusses the efficacy of antibiotic regimens and novel therapies in treating commonly encountered multidrug-resistant organisms.

When the terms funguria or fungal urinary tract infection are used, most physicians are referring to candiduria and urinary tract infections due to *Candida* species. Other fungi, including yeasts and molds can involve the kidney during the course of disseminated infection, but rarely cause symptoms referable to the urinary tract. *Candida* species appear to be unique in their ability to both colonize and cause invasive disease in the urinary tract. This overview focuses only on candiduria and *Candida* urinary tract infection because they are common and many times present perplexing management issues.

Urinary tract infection (UTI) is a commonly diagnosed infection in older adults. Despite consensus guidelines developed to assist providers in diagnosing UTI, distinguishing symptomatic UTI from asymptomatic bacteriuria (ASB) in older adults is problematic, as many older adults do not present with localized genitourinary symptoms. This article summarizes the recent literature and guidelines on the diagnosis and management of UTI and ASB in older adults.

Some populations have unique considerations relevant to complicated urinary tract infection. For patients with diabetes, renal transplant, HIV infection, and spinal cord injuries, approaches to management, including diagnosis and treatment, are generally similar to other patients with complicated urinary tract infection. In addition, there is no evidence that treatment of asymptomatic bacteriuria leads to improved outcomes.

Catheter-associated urinary tract infection (CAUTI) is common, costly, and causes significant patient morbidity. CAUTIs are associated with hospital pathogens with a high propensity toward antimicrobial resistance. Treatment of asymptomatic patients with CAUTI accounts for excess antimicrobial use in hospitals and should be avoided. Duration of urinary catheterization is the predominant risk for CAUTI; preventive measures directed at limiting placement and early removal of urinary catheters have an impact on decreasing CAUTI rates. The use of bladder bundles and collaboratives, coupled with the support and active engagement from both hospital leaders and followers, seem to help prevent this common problem.

This article presents an overview of non-catheter-associated complicated urinary tract infection (UTI) from a urologic point of view. Discussion includes the evaluation and workup of complicated UTI through history, physical examination, laboratory analysis, and radiographic studies. Specific types of complicated UTI, such as urinary obstruction and renal abscess, are reviewed.

Recurrent urinary tract infections (UTIs) are common, especially in women. Low-dose daily or postcoital antimicrobial prophylaxis is effective for prevention of recurrent UTIs and women can self-diagnose and self-treat a new UTI with antibiotics. The increasing resistance rates of *Escherichia coli* to antimicrobial agents has, however, stimulated interest in nonantibiotic methods for the prevention of UTIs. This article reviews the literature on efficacy of different forms of nonantibiotic prophylaxis. Future studies with lactobacilli strains (oral and vaginal) and the oral immunostimulant OM-89 are warranted.

Clinically, host factors in the pathogenesis of urinary tract infection (UTI) may be considered as modifiable (eg, behaviors associated with increased risk of UTI, anatomic and functional problems of the urinary tract) and thus potentially amenable to a change in patient behavior or treatment approach, or as intrinsic and nonmodifiable host factors that neither the patient nor the clinician can influence (eg, gender and genetic influences associated with UTI). Although considering nonmodifiable host factors may be discouraging to patients and clinicians at present, some genetic associations have the potential for future predictive value and may interface with future treatments.

INFECTIOUS DISEASE CLINICS
OF NORTH AMERICA

RELATED INTEREST

Primary Care: Clinics in Office Practice, September 2013 (Vol. 40, Issue 3)
Infectious Disease
Michael A. Malone, *Editor*
Available at: http://www.primarycare.theclinics.com/

DOWNLOAD
Free App!

Review Articles
THE CLINICS

NOW AVAILABLE FOR YOUR iPhone and iPad

Preface

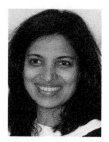

Kalpana Gupta, MD, MPH
Editor

It has been over a decade since the last *Infectious Disease Clinics of North America* issue dedicated to UTI was published. During this time, the approach to this broad clinical syndrome has been impacted by ever-increasing antibacterial resistance, political and financial ramifications, and an evolving understanding about the role of the human microbiome in the prevention of infectious diseases.

In this issue, well-recognized experts have contributed articles aimed at optimizing the diagnosis, management, and prevention of UTI. The infection remains exceedingly common, being one of the primary reasons for an emergency room visit made by otherwise healthy women. The risk factors and burden of disease vary by patient population and the specific urinary tract syndrome. Characterization of the specific syndrome remains important for appropriate diagnosis and management.

The concept of asymptomatic bacteriuria and candiduria as conditions not warranting therapy in most situations is increasingly being accepted and incorporated into clinical practice guidelines and stewardship programs. The diagnosis of UTI in the hospital setting, especially in patients with urinary catheters, has taken on new significance in the past several years. Prevention of catheter-associated UTI is now a Joint Commission National Patient Safety Goal, making accurate diagnosis of infection versus colonization a critical issue. In addition, hospitals are no longer reimbursed for catheter-associated UTIs that occur in the hospital, and rates are being publically reported in some cases, creating political and financial pressures to reduce these infections.

Appropriate management of UTI in different patient care settings including primary care, the emergency department, and acute and long-term care inpatient settings is becoming more challenging. Resistance among uropathogens is now not only an issue for complicated hospital-associated UTIs, but for simple community-acquired infections as well. With rising resistance across multiple classes of drugs, oral options for UTI are limited and sometimes nonexistent. Choosing an empiric oral therapy regimen that is likely to be active for outpatient cystitis is necessitating the use of older drugs such as nitrofurantoin and fosfomycin rather than the more familiar sulfa- and fluoroquinolone classes of agents. Oral options for more invasive UTI are even further

Infect Dis Clin N Am 28 (2014) ix–x
http://dx.doi.org/10.1016/j.idc.2013.11.001
0891-5520/14/$ – see front matter © 2014 Published by Elsevier Inc.

constrained, resulting in the need for intravenous therapy for infections that have traditionally been managed in the outpatient setting.

Prevention of infection and judicious use of antimicrobials are concepts that have come to the forefront and directly impact the management of UTI. Non-antimicrobial approaches to prevention are being prioritized over the traditional use of suppressive antibiotics by some patients because avoiding antibiotics and sparing the gut microbiome is now recognized as a desirable benefit outweighing the potential risk of lower efficacy. Understanding of the pathogenesis of UTI has also evolved; both microbiological and genomics-based studies demonstrate the importance of Lactobacillus spp in the vaginal microbiota. Therapeutic interventions to address alterations in the urogenital microbiota and prevent UTI are currently being studied.

Thus, the overall approach to diagnosis and management of UTI has markedly shifted in the past decade. I am grateful to the editors of the *Infectious Disease Clinics of North America* for giving me the opportunity to serve as guest editor and to the distinguished group of colleagues who have contributed their expertise to make this issue an informative and valuable resource for years to come.

Kalpana Gupta, MD, MPH
Infectious Diseases
VA Boston HCS
West Roxbury, MA, USA

Infectious Diseases
Boston University School of Medicine
Boston, MA, USA

E-mail address:
Kalpana.Gupta@va.gov

Urinary Tract Infection Syndromes
Occurrence, Recurrence, Bacteriology, Risk Factors, and Disease Burden

Betsy Foxman, PhD

KEYWORDS

- Asymptomatic bacteriuria • Cystitis • Pyelonephritis
- Catheter-associated urinary tract infection

KEY POINTS

- The bladder is continuously invaded by bacteria, which can grow to substantial numbers before spontaneous clearance.
- Host factors, host behaviors, and bacterial characteristics are risk factors for the development of symptoms.
- Urinary tract infection (UTI) occurs more often in females than in males.
- Except during pregnancy, asymptomatic bacteriuria is not a treatable condition.
- Cystitis and pyelonephritis are likely to recur, regardless of age, gender, or treatment.
- The gram-negative rod *Escherichia coli* is the most common cause of UTI in all settings, and is transmitted by person-to-person direct contact and the fecal-oral route.
- The proportion of UTI caused by species other than *E coli* is higher in recurring UTI and hospital-acquired UTI.
- The urinary tract is the most common source of bacteremia caused by *E coli*.

DISEASE DESCRIPTION

Urinary tract infection (UTI), an infection anywhere in the urinary tract (urethra, bladder, ureters, or kidneys) is very common. In 2007 in the United States there were 10.5 million ambulatory visits for UTI, accounting for 0.9% of all ambulatory visits.[1] Almost one-fifth (21.3%) of these visits were to hospital emergency departments. UTI is among the most common primary diagnoses for United States women visiting emergency departments.[2] Prevalence of UTI is high among inpatients also: in a 2004 survey of symptomatic UTI among 49 Swiss hospitals, UTI was detected in 3.7% of those who had been catheterized for at least 24 hours during their hospital stay, and in 0.9% of those who had not been catheterized.[3]

The author declares no conflicts of interest.
Department of Epidemiology, University of Michigan School of Public Health, 1415 Washington Heights, Ann Arbor, MI 48109-2029, USA
E-mail address: bfoxman@umich.edu

Infect Dis Clin N Am 28 (2014) 1–13
http://dx.doi.org/10.1016/j.idc.2013.09.003
0891-5520/14/$ – see front matter © 2014 Elsevier Inc. All rights reserved.

id.theclinics.com

This review defines the major UTI syndromes (**Table 1**), their occurrence and recurrence, bacteriology, risk factors, and disease burden. Although the bacteria that cause UTI are increasingly resistant to antibiotic therapies (reviewed elsewhere in this issue), and modern molecular techniques have made it possible to better characterize the genetic lineages of uropathogens, UTI occurrence and risk factors, with few exceptions, have remained relatively constant.

UTI SYNDROMES AND THEIR OCCURRENCE: ASYMPTOMATIC BACTERIURIA, CYSTITIS, PYELONEPHRITIS, AND CATHETER-ASSOCIATED UTI

The urinary tract has a portal to the outside, making it particularly susceptible to invasion by microbes. Bacteria normally inhabit the tissues around the urethral opening, and frequently colonize the urine. Among men, culture of a random initial void will find 1% to 5% colonized with *Escherichia coli*; urethral colonization is higher among men whose female sex partner has a UTI.[4] Among women, urinary colonization rates are higher; the vaginal cavity and rectal opening are close to the urethral opening, and women have more moist periurethral areas where bacteria grow. On entering the urethra, the bacteria are more likely to ascend to the female bladder than the male bladder because of the shorter urethral length. The overall prevalence of asymptomatic bacteriuria (ASB) in women is 3.5%,[5] but is much higher following sexual intercourse.[6] Among both men and women, the prevalence of asymptomatic bacteriuria increases with age.[5,7] Laboratory findings for ASB are the same as for other UTI syndromes (ie, a positive urine culture and urinalysis), but there are no signs or symptoms referable to the urinary tract (**Table 1**).

With the exception of during pregnancy, ASB is not a treatable condition. Treatment of ASB in the otherwise healthy individual often results in a symptomatic UTI,[8] and increases selection for antibiotic-resistant bacteria. The Infectious Disease Society of America recommends against screening for and treating ASB among catheterized patients.[9] However, physiologic changes during pregnancy make the

Table 1
Urinary tract infection syndromes: laboratory findings, signs, and symptoms

Syndrome	Laboratory Findings		Signs and Symptoms
	Culture	Urinalysis	
Asymptomatic bacteriuria (ASB)	+	+	None referable to urinary tract
Cystitis	+	+	Frequency, urgency, dysuria; less commonly suprapubic pressure, malaise, nocturia, incontinence (more common in children and elderly)
Pyelonephritis	+	+	Frequency, urgency, dysuria, back pain, flank pain, fever, chills, malaise, nausea, vomiting, anorexia, abdominal pain
Catheter-associated UTI	+	+	Fever, chills, altered mental state, malaise or lethargy with no other identified cause; flank pain, costovertebral angle tenderness, acute hematuria, pelvic discomfort. If catheter has been removed: same as for cystitis or pyelonephritis

pregnant woman with ASB more susceptible to pyelonephritis.[10] The prevalence of ASB in pregnancy ranges from 2% to 20%; and one-fifth to two-fifths of these may develop pyelonephritis if untreated.[11] Pyelonephritis can be life threatening to both the mother and infant.[11] Screening and treating ASB during pregnancy may reduce this risk by 77%.[12]

The high frequency of ASB does complicate the diagnosis of UTI, as urinary symptoms considered enigmatic of UTI, namely frequency, urgency and dysuria, are not solely caused by UTI. Vaginitis, chlamydia, and gonorrhea also cause urinary symptoms. Therefore, the chance of ASB and urinary symptoms occurring together by chance alone is not insignificant, especially as these conditions are also associated with sexual activity. By contrast, up to half of women at high risk of UTI (sexually active women aged 18–29 years) with frequency, urgency, and dysuria will have a negative urine culture when the limit of detection is 1000 cfu/mL urine.[13,14]

In cystitis, urinary symptoms are confined to the bladder, although upper tract involvement occurs. Among premenopausal women, frequency, urgency, and dysuria are the most common symptoms. Among postmenopausal women, the elderly, and children, the patient may present with malaise, nocturia, incontinence, or a complaint of foul-smelling urine (see **Table 1**). Cystitis is very common. For example, among veteran users of the Veterans' Administration health care, the annual incidence was 4.3% among women and 1.7% among men.[15] This figure is similar to population-based estimates from the Calgary Health Region of Canada, where the annual incidence of community-onset UTI identified using laboratory surveillance was 3% for females and 0.5% for males.[16] Estimates based on self-reported history of physician diagnosis during the past year are higher: approximately 12.6% per year for women and 3.0% per year for men.[17] Estimated lifetime risk of UTI for women based on self-reported history of physician diagnosis is 60.4%.[18]

Urinary symptoms may or may not be present in pyelonephritis; the patient may present with fever and chills, back pain, nausea, and vomiting (see **Table 1**). The incidence of pyelonephritis is an order of magnitude lower than cystitis (59.0/10,000 for females and 12.6/10,000 for males), but the patterns by age and sex are very similar.[19] Risks are higher for females than for males, but these differences decrease with age (**Fig. 1**). In the United States, the incidence of hospitalization for acute pyelonephritis is 11.7 in 10,000 for women and 2.4 in 10,000 for men.[20] A population-based study in California estimated the incidence of hospitalization for pyelonephritis among children to be 31 in 100,000 in 2005. The incidence varied substantially by age, with children younger than 1 year having the highest rates.[21]

Every day that a urinary catheter is in place increases the risk of bacteriuria by 3% to 10%.[22] However, unless there are symptoms referable to the urinary tract or there are generalized symptoms such as fever, chills, or malaise with no identifiable cause (see **Table 1**), catheter-associated bacteriuria is not a treatable condition.[9] Catheters are the major risk factor for hospital-acquired UTI, which account for almost one-third of all hospital-acquired infections. The estimated rates of catheter-associated UTI vary by service: in an analysis of 15 hospitals in the Duke Infection Control Outreach Network, the rates were 1.83 per 1000 catheter days for patients in intensive care, compared with 1.55 per 1000 catheter days for other patients.[23] The risk of UTI with catheterization varies only slightly by catheter type. A multicenter, randomized controlled trial in the United Kingdom compared antimicrobial-impregnated, antiseptic-coated (silver alloy), and standard polytetrafluoroethylene-coated catheters in 7102 participants. Incidence of UTI any time up to 6 weeks following randomization in the 3 groups ranged from 10.6% to 12.6%, and was not significantly different between the groups.[24]

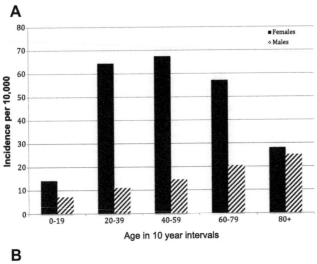

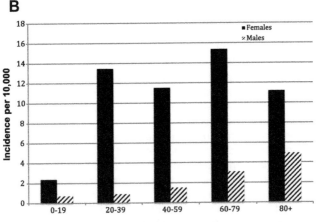

Fig. 1. Annual incidence of pyelonephritis per 10,000, by sex. (*A*) Pyelonephritis treated as outpatients. (*B*) Pyelonephritis treated in hospital. Data are taken from South Korean insurance claims, 1997 to 1999. (*Adapted from* Ki M, Park T, Choi B, et al. The epidemiology of acute pyelonephritis in South Korea, 1997–1999. Am J Epidemiol 2004;160:988; with permission.)

RECURRENCE

UTI has a propensity to recur with a frequency that varies by population (**Table 2**). Among children younger than 16 years with UTI participating in UTI intervention trials in Australia and Finland, the risk of recurrence within 1 year was 19% to 22%.[25,26] The risk of recurrence is even higher among sexually active young women. In a Michigan study following 285 college women with first UTI for 6 months, the risk of a second was 24% within 6 months.[27] In a Seattle study of 796 women starting a new method of contraception, the risk of first UTI was 0.5 per person-year among college students and 0.3 per person-year among participants enrolled at a health maintenance organization.[28] Also in the Seattle study, women with a history of 2 or more UTIs compared

Table 2		
Risk of recurrence by urinary syndrome and age group		
Age Group	UTI	Pyelonephritis
Children	19%–22% within 5 y	21% within 5 y
Women	30%–50% per year	9% per year
Men	12% per year	6% per year

with those with only 1 or no UTI history had 2 to 5 times the risk of recurrence within a year.[28] A similar pattern is seen in postmenopausal women with a history of 3 of more UTIs in the previous year. In a Dutch double-blind noninferiority trial that included 252 postmenopausal women, 69.3% of those assigned to daily trimethoprim-sulfamethoxazole had recurrence of UTI within 12 months, compared with 79.1% assigned to lactobacilli prophylaxis. The mean number of recurrences in the 12-month follow-up period was 2.9 and 3.3, respectively.[29] UTI in men also has a tendency to recur. Among male veterans treated as outpatients for UTI at the Veteran Affairs system, the risk of recurrence within 30 days was 4.1%. Recurrence within 31 to 364 days occurred in 8.1%.[30]

Pyelonephritis also recurs. In a Tennessee study, 21% of children with a first episode of pyelonephritis between the ages of 2 and 24 months had a second episode within 5 years.[31] This finding was true even among children with normal ultrasonograms and voiding cystourethrograms: a New York retrospective telephone follow-up study of 119 children with a first UTI before 6 months of age with normal radiography found a recurrence rate of 20% by age 5 years.[32] Among adults in South Korea, the 12-month risk of recurrence was 9.2% for females and 5.7% for males. However, risk of subsequent recurrences was substantially higher: 21.7% for a second recurrence to 53% for a fifth recurrence for females, and 21.6% for a second recurrence and 50% for a fifth recurrence for males.[19]

BACTERIOLOGY

Urine is a good medium for bacterial growth, so it is not surprising that many bacteria can grow in the urinary tract, and do so frequently (**Box 1**, **Fig. 2**). The bacteria colonizing the urinary tract do not cause disease in most cases because the host has many effective methods for rapidly removing bacteria from the system. These methods include urination and innate and adaptive host immune response. Bacteria that do cause UTI either have special features that enable them to survive in the urinary tract (eg, biofilm formation, urothelial cell invasion,[33] adhesins, toxins, and siderophores)[34] or inhabit a host that is compromised in a way that limits their ability to remove bacteria (eg, a catheter is in place). This fact explains the higher rate of UTI

Box 1
Bacteriology

- *Escherichia coli* causes the majority of asymptomatic bacteriuria, cystitis, pyelonephritis, and catheter-associated urinary tract infection (UTI)

- The proportion of UTI caused by species other than *Escherichia coli* is higher in recurring UTI and hospital-acquired UTI

- Antibiotic resistance is increasing, but patterns of resistance vary with patient population and geographic region

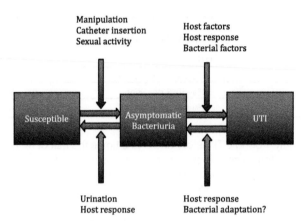

Manipulation
Catheter insertion
Sexual activity

Host factors
Host response
Bacterial factors

Susceptible

Asymptomatic
Bacteriuria

UTI

Urination
Host response

Host response
Bacterial adaptation?

Fig. 2. Model of urinary tract infection syndromes.

among hospitalized patients: the prevalence of UTI on any 1 day among hospitalized patients is 1.1% to 6.5%; among those without urinary catheters or any exposure to urinary catheters, the point prevalence is 0.9%.[3] By comparison, estimates for cystitis in the community are 0.5% to 3% per year for males and 3% to 12.6% per year for females.[16,17]

E coli causes the majority of infections in all settings, for all syndromes and all age groups: 74.4% among outpatients regardless of age group, 65% of hospital-acquired infections, and 47% of health care–associated infections.[16] The *E coli* that cause UTI are remarkably diverse, varying in the presence of known uropathogenic factors,[35,36] and represent multiple different genetic lineages.[37,38] Although the antibiotic resistances of uropathogenic *E coli* have increased over the past 30 years, resistance patterns are variable, depending on patient population and geographic region.[39]

In addition to *E coli*, species that cause UTI, with varying frequency, are the gram-negative *Klebsiella* spp, *Pseudomonas aeruginosa*, and *Proteus* spp, and the gram-positive *Streptococcus agalactiae* and *Staphylococcus saprophyticus*. Individuals with recurrent UTI, males, those with a foreign body or obstruction, or with a urinary catheter, are more likely to have a UTI attributable to non–*E coli*.[40]

RISK FACTORS

Risk factors for UTI (**Box 2**) can be divided into factors that expose the host to potential uropathogens, those that enhance colonization by the uropathogens, and those that lead the host to respond to colonization causing diseases (see **Fig. 2**). Uropathogens live in multiple environments, including the bowel, periurethral area, vaginal cavity, and urinary tract; they are transferred between individuals via person-to-person direct contact, including sexual activity, and via the fecal-oral route. Most uropathogens have special features that enable them to inhabit the urinary tract (see the section on bacteriology).

Bacteria found in the bowel, periurethral area, and vaginal cavity constantly move into the urinary tract. This movement is enhanced by manipulation, catheter insertion, and sexual activity. Females are particularly susceptible, because of the shorter distance between the urethral and anal opening and vaginal cavity, where potential uropathogens live. The distance from the urethral opening to the bladder is also shorter in

Box 2
Risk factors
• Female sex
• Prior UTI
• Sexual activity
• Condom/diaphragm/spermicide use
• Vaginal infection
• Trauma/manipulation
• Diabetes
• Obesity
• Genetic susceptibility/anatomic abnormalities

females, making it easier for bacteria to ascend into the bladder, and females have more moist areas in the periurethrum where bacteria grow. However, symptoms only occur when the host response is engaged; the chances of immune-response engagement increase in those who are unable to urinate frequently, empty their bladder completely (such as those with neurogenic bladder or with obstruction), or are immunocompromised (those with comorbidities and increased age). ASB is generally transient, but some individuals are colonized for extended periods.[41] Even when ASB is transient, uropathogens grow to substantial numbers (>100,000 cfu/mL urine), facilitating transmission to new hosts, some of whom may develop symptoms.

As noted earlier, UTI have a tendency to recur. A history of a previous UTI is a major risk factor for UTI. Whether this is a function of host behavior, host susceptibility, bacterial factors, or an interaction of the 3 is unclear. Host behavior is strongly associated with UTI. Sexual activity moves bacteria into the urethra in both males and females, increasing the risk for UTI. College women with their first UTI were 21 times more likely than controls to have engaged in vaginal intercourse 1 to 5 times during the previous 2 weeks.[42] Condoms, diaphragms, and spermicide also are associated with an increase in UTI risk. Condom use may increase trauma; the increased risk associated with condom use is somewhat ameliorated by lubricant use.[43] A diaphragm may obstruct urine flow; there is also an independent effect of spermicide use on UTI risk, and spermicides are generally used with diaphragms.[27] Vaginal infections, such as bacterial vaginosis,[44,45] can facilitate the growth of E coli, which probably accounts for their association with increased risk for UTI. Risk factors for pyelonephritis among otherwise healthy women are essentially the same as risk factors for cystitis.[46] Pregnant women are at higher risk of pyelonephritis, because of anatomic changes that occur during pregnancy.[10]

Placement of a catheter moves bacteria into the bladder, and creates an additional portal for bacterial invasion; catheter placement increases the risk of UTI by as much as 4-fold.[3] However, any manipulation and presence of comorbidities increases UTI risk. In the United States, estimates of the point prevalence of UTI (based on the National Nursing Home Survey and National Home and Hospice Care Survey) are 5.2% among nursing home residents, 3.6% among those receiving home health care, and 3% of those receiving hospice care. UTI was the most common infection among those surveyed in all 3 sites.[47] Undergoing surgery for any reason greatly increases UTI risk, especially if it involves manipulation of the genitourinary tract and placement of a urinary catheter. Overall, UTI incidence in the 30 days following surgery is 1.7%, but is

2.6% among patients undergoing nonalimentary and noncolorectal tract surgery (95% confidence interval [CI] 2.2%–2.9%), compared with 5.6% (95% CI 4.6%–6.8%) for those undergoing abdominoperineal resection.[48] Risk of UTI following surgery for incontinence is substantially higher: in the 6 weeks following surgery, the incidence is reported to range from 10% to 32%.[49,50]

The risk of UTI increases with age. The annual incidence of UTI among very old women in Sweden (85 years and older) was 29.6%. In this group, risk factors included vertebral fractures, incontinence, inflammatory rheumatic disease, and multi-infarct dementia.[51] In the Leiden 85-Plus Study, the incidence of UTI among women was 12.8 per 100 person-years, and 7.8 per 100 person-years among men. The strongest predictors of UTI risk were severe cognitive impairment, disability in daily living, recent history of UTI, and urinary incontinence.[52]

Type 2 diabetes also increases the risk of UTI. In a United Kingdom study conducted using the General Practice Research Database, younger men aged 18 to 39 years with diabetes were more than 4 times more likely to have UTI than their peers without diabetes.[53] The risk was also somewhat higher among individuals whose diabetes was poorly controlled. Overall, the adjusted relative risk of UTI among females with diabetes was 1.53 (95% CI 1.45–1.60), and 1.49 (95% CI 1.38–1.60) for males with diabetes (estimates adjusted for age and prior history of UTI). Obesity is a risk factor for diabetes, and also has been reported as a risk factor for UTI. A study conducted using insurees of the largest not-for-profit health care provider in Israel examined the joint association of obesity and diabetes on UTI risk. Unfortunately, this study did not take into account UTI history. After adjusting for age, body mass index (BMI), and vitamin D level, which is associated with increased risk of infection, diabetes increased the risk of UTI by 23% in males 24% in females. However, obesity was independently associated with UTI after adjustment for age, diabetes, and vitamin D levels: males with BMI of 50 kg/m^2 or higher were 2.38 (95% CI 1.40–4.03) times more likely than those with a BMI of less than 25 kg/m^2 to have a UTI; for females the increased risk was 1.25 (95% CI 1.03–1.52) (**Fig. 3**).[54] Because the United Kingdom and Israeli study were conducted using medical records, they were unable

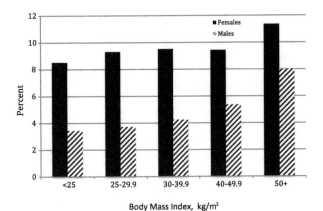

Fig. 3. Annual incidence of urinary tract infection per 100, by sex and body mass index. Individuals aged 18 years and older insured by the largest not-for-profit health care provider in Israel, 2009 to 2012. (*Adapted from* Saliba W, Barnett-Griness O, Rennert G. The association between obesity and urinary tract infection. Eur J Intern Med 2013;24:128; with permission.)

to adjust for sexual activity (see the article by Nicolle elsewhere in this issue for further discussion of diabetes and the risk of UTI).

Some individuals seem to be more inherently susceptible to UTI. Part of this susceptibility may be attributed to host behaviors such as frequency of sexual activity and urination habits. However, there is increasing evidence of genetic susceptibility. Women with recurrent cystitis and pyelonephritis are more likely than age-matched controls with no UTI history to report their female relatives as having a history of UTI.[55] This finding suggests that there might be a genetic component, but it is difficult with this study design to rule out the possibility that women with recurring UTI might be more likely to know their family history. Stronger evidence derives from studies demonstrating polymorphisms in genes coding for inflammatory response (toll-like receptors, interferon regulatory factors, and chemokine receptors) between individuals with ASB and pyelonephritis.[56,57] However, it is most likely that variation in disease severity results from an interaction between bacterial virulence genes and host response.[58]

DISEASE BURDEN

The vast majority of UTIs are confined to the bladder (**Box 3**). Typical symptoms are hematuria, dysuria, urgency, frequency, nocturia, offensive smell, and abdominal pain. In a study of 684 women aged 18 to 70 years with UTI, participants reported an average of 3.83 symptom days, 2.89 restricted-activity days, and 3.13 days during which they were unwell. Most symptoms lasted no more than 3 days, with hematuria having the shortest duration (1.88 days) and urinary frequency the longest (3.14 days).[59] The risk that cystitis will progress to pyelonephritis is low, less than 1% (reviewed in Ref.[60]), although a recent UTI does increase the risk of pyelonephritis by 4.4 times (95% CI 2.8–7.10); note that women with pyelonephritis were 5.6 times more likely than controls to engage in sexual intercourse 3 or more times per week. The estimated annual direct and indirect cost of UTI in the United States is $2.3 billion in 2010 dollars.[60]

Acute pyelonephritis among adults results in hospitalization for 10% to 30% of patients. The direct and indirect costs were estimated as $2.14 billion in 2000 (which is ~$2.9 billion in 2013).[20] Patients with acute pyelonephritis are increasingly managed as outpatients, greatly reducing costs.[61] However, with increasing antibiotic resistance, the need for intravenous administration of antibiotics—and hospital admission—may increase. Pyelonephritis in pregnancy can cause serious morbidity. In a study conducted using a Nationwide Inpatient Sample in 2006, pregnant patients hospitalized for pyelonephritis stayed a mean of 2.8 days, for an estimated annual cost of $263 million in 2012 dollars. Although the risk of death was very low, almost 2% had sepsis, 0.77% had acute respiratory failure, and 3.77% had threatened preterm labor.[62]

The urinary tract is a frequent source of bacteremia, and the urinary tract is the most common source of *E coli* bacteremia. In Olmstead County the age-adjusted incidence of gram-negative bacteremic UTI was 55.3 per 100,000 for females and 44.6 per

---

Box 3
Disease burden

- Women with UTI average 3.83 symptom days and 2.89 restricted-activity days
- Risk of cystitis progressing to pyelonephritis is less than 1%
- Urinary tract is the most common source of *E coli* bacteremia

100,000 for males. Risk of bacteremia increased sharply at ages 60 to 79, and exceeded 4 per 1000 among those 80 and older, among whom the risks were higher in males than in females. The mortality rate after 28 days for any cause was 4.9%.[63] Risk factors for bacteremia among inpatients identified in a Missouri study of 156 patients with *E coli* bacteriuria at the time of admission included benign prostatic hyperplasia, a history of urogenital surgery, pyelonephritis, and presentation with hesitancy/retention or fever.[64]

The risk of bacteremia and subsequent mortality is substantially higher among inpatients with urinary catheters. In a United Kingdom study of 559 bacteremic episodes among 437 patients, almost 15% were associated with urinary catheters, second only to bacteremia associated with central venous catheters.[65] Among those with catheter-associated bacteremic UTI, the risk of mortality within 7 days was 30.1%.[65]

SUMMARY

- The bladder is continuously invaded by bacteria, which can grow to substantial numbers before spontaneous clearance.
- Host factors, host behaviors, and bacterial characteristics are risk factors for the development of symptoms.
- UTI occurs more often in females than in males.
- Except during pregnancy, ASB is not a treatable condition.
- Cystitis and pyelonephritis are likely to recur, regardless of age, gender, or treatment.
- The gram-negative rod *E coli* is the most common cause of UTI in all settings, and is transmitted by person-to-person direct contact and the fecal-oral route.
- The proportion of UTI caused by species other than *E coli* is higher in recurring UTI and hospital-acquired UTI.
- The urinary tract is the most common source of bacteremia attributable to *E coli*.

REFERENCES

1. Schappert SM, Rechtsteiner EA. Ambulatory medical care utilization estimates for 2007. Vital Health Stat 13 2011;(169):1–38.
2. Niska R, Bhuiya F, Xu J. National hospital ambulatory medical care survey: 2007 emergency department summary. Natl Health Stat Report 2010;(26):1–31.
3. Uckay I, Sax H, Gayet-Ageron A, et al. High proportion of healthcare-associated urinary tract infection in the absence of prior exposure to urinary catheter: a cross-sectional study. Antimicrob Resist Infect Control 2013;2:5.
4. Foxman B, Manning SD, Tallman P, et al. Uropathogenic *Escherichia coli* are more likely than commensal *E. coli* to be shared between heterosexual sex partners. Am J Epidemiol 2002;156:1133–40.
5. Evans DA, Williams DN, Laughlin LW, et al. Bacteriuria in a population-based cohort of women. J Infect Dis 1978;138:768–73.
6. Nicolle LE, Harding GK, Preiksaitis J, et al. The association of urinary tract infection with sexual intercourse. J Infect Dis 1982;146:579–83.
7. Nicolle LE. Urinary tract infections in the elderly. Clin Geriatr Med 2009;25: 423–36.
8. Cai T, Mazzoli S, Mondaini N, et al. The role of asymptomatic bacteriuria in young women with recurrent urinary tract infections: to treat or not to treat? Clin Infect Dis 2012;55:771–7.
9. Hooton TM, Bradley SF, Cardenas DD, et al. Diagnosis, prevention, and treatment of catheter-associated urinary tract infection in adults: 2009 International

Clinical Practice Guidelines from the Infectious Diseases Society of America. Clin Infect Dis 2010;50:625–63.

10. Ramos NL, Sekikubo M, Dzung DT, et al. Uropathogenic *Escherichia coli* isolates from pregnant women in different countries. J Clin Microbiol 2012;50:3569–74.

11. Kazemier BM, Schneeberger C, De Miranda E, et al. Costs and effects of screening and treating low risk women with a singleton pregnancy for asymptomatic bacteriuria, the ASB study. BMC Pregnancy Childbirth 2012;12:52.

12. Smaill F, Vazquez JC. Antibiotics for asymptomatic bacteriuria in pregnancy. Cochrane Database Syst Rev 2007;(2):CD000490.

13. Gordon LB, Waxman MJ, Ragsdale L, et al. Overtreatment of presumed urinary tract infection in older women presenting to the emergency department. J Am Geriatr Soc 2013;61:788–92.

14. Bent S, Nallamothu BK, Simel DL, et al. Does this woman have an acute uncomplicated urinary tract infection? JAMA 2002;287:2701–10.

15. Anger JT, Saigal CS, Wang M, et al. Urologic disease burden in the United States: veteran users of Department of Veterans Affairs healthcare. Urology 2008;72:37–41 [discussion: 41].

16. Laupland KB, Ross T, Pitout JD, et al. Community-onset urinary tract infections: a population-based assessment. Infection 2007;35:150–3.

17. Foxman B, Brown P. Epidemiology of urinary tract infections: transmission and risk factors, incidence, and costs. Infect Dis Clin North Am 2003;17:227–41.

18. Foxman B, Barlow R, D'Arcy H, et al. Urinary tract infection: self-reported incidence and associated costs. Ann Epidemiol 2000;10:509–15.

19. Ki M, Park T, Choi B, et al. The epidemiology of acute pyelonephritis in South Korea, 1997-1999. Am J Epidemiol 2004;160:985–93.

20. Brown P, Ki M, Foxman B. Acute pyelonephritis among adults: cost of illness and considerations for the economic evaluation of therapy. Pharmacoeconomics 2005;23:1123–42.

21. Copp HL, Halpern MS, Maldonado Y, et al. Trends in hospitalization for pediatric pyelonephritis: a population based study of California from 1985 to 2006. J Urol 2011;186:1028–34.

22. Warren JW, Platt R, Thomas RJ, et al. Antibiotic irrigation and catheter-associated urinary-tract infections. N Engl J Med 1978;299:570–3.

23. Lewis SS, Knelson LP, Moehring RW, et al. Comparison of non-intensive care unit (ICU) versus ICU rates of catheter-associated urinary tract infection in community hospitals. Infect Control Hosp Epidemiol 2013;34:744–7.

24. Pickard R, Lam T, Maclennan G, et al. Types of urethral catheter for reducing symptomatic urinary tract infections in hospitalised adults requiring short-term catheterisation: multicentre randomised controlled trial and economic evaluation of antimicrobial- and antiseptic-impregnated urethral catheters (the CATHETER trial). Health Technol Assess 2012;16:1–197.

25. Craig JC, Simpson JM, Williams GJ, et al. Antibiotic prophylaxis and recurrent urinary tract infection in children. N Engl J Med 2009;361:1748–59.

26. Salo J, Uhari M, Helminen M, et al. Cranberry juice for the prevention of recurrences of urinary tract infections in children: a randomized placebo-controlled trial. Clin Infect Dis 2012;54:340–6.

27. Foxman B, Gillespie B, Koopman J, et al. Risk factors for second urinary tract infection among college women. Am J Epidemiol 2000;151:1194–205.

28. Hooton TM, Scholes D, Hughes JP, et al. A prospective study of risk factors for symptomatic urinary tract infection in young women. N Engl J Med 1996;335:468–74.

29. Beerepoot MA, ter Riet G, Nys S, et al. Lactobacilli vs antibiotics to prevent urinary tract infections: a randomized, double-blind, noninferiority trial in postmenopausal women. Arch Intern Med 2012;172:704–12.

30. Drekonja DM, Rector TS, Cutting A, et al. Urinary tract infection in male veterans: treatment patterns and outcomes. JAMA Intern Med 2013;173:62–8.

31. Juliano TM, Stephany HA, Clayton DB, et al. Incidence of abnormal imaging and recurrent pyelonephritis after first febrile urinary tract infection in children 2 to 24 months old. J Urol 2013;190(Suppl 4):1505–10.

32. Bratslavsky G, Feustel PJ, Aslan AR, et al. Recurrence risk in infants with urinary tract infections and a negative radiographic evaluation. J Urol 2004;172:1610–3 [discussion: 1613].

33. Mulvey MA, Schilling JD, Martinez JJ, et al. Bad bugs and beleaguered bladders: interplay between uropathogenic *Escherichia coli* and innate host defenses. Proc Natl Acad Sci U S A 2000;97:8829–35.

34. Pitout JD. Extraintestinal pathogenic *Escherichia coli*: a combination of virulence with antibiotic resistance. Front Microbiol 2012;3:9.

35. Marrs CF, Zhang L, Foxman B. *Escherichia coli* mediated urinary tract infections: are there distinct uropathogenic *E. coli* (UPEC) pathotypes? FEMS Microbiol Lett 2005;252:183–90.

36. Vigil PD, Stapleton AE, Johnson JR, et al. Presence of putative repeat-in-toxin gene tosA in *Escherichia coli* predicts successful colonization of the urinary tract. MBio 2011;2. e00066–11.

37. Poulsen HO, Johansson A, Granholm S, et al. High genetic diversity of nitrofurantoin- or mecillinam-resistant *Escherichia coli* indicates low propensity for clonal spread. J Antimicrob Chemother 2013;68(9):1974–7.

38. Wirth T, Falush D, Lan R, et al. Sex and virulence in *Escherichia coli*: an evolutionary perspective. Mol Microbiol 2006;60:1136–51.

39. Kahlmeter G, Poulsen HO. Antimicrobial susceptibility of *Escherichia coli* from community-acquired urinary tract infections in Europe: the ECO SENS study revisited. Int J Antimicrob Agents 2012;39:45–51.

40. Amna MA, Chazan B, Raz R, et al. Risk factors for non-*Escherichia coli* community-acquired bacteriuria. Infection 2013;41:473–7.

41. Salvador E, Wagenlehner F, Kohler CD, et al. Comparison of asymptomatic bacteriuria *Escherichia coli* isolates from healthy individuals versus those from hospital patients shows that long-term bladder colonization selects for attenuated virulence phenotypes. Infect Immun 2012;80:668–78.

42. Foxman B, Geiger AM, Palin K, et al. First-time urinary tract infection and sexual behavior. Epidemiology 1995;6:162–8.

43. Foxman B, Marsh J, Gillespie B, et al. Condom use and first-time urinary tract infection. Epidemiology 1997;8:637–41.

44. Hillebrand L, Harmanli OH, Whiteman V, et al. Urinary tract infections in pregnant women with bacterial vaginosis. Am J Obstet Gynecol 2002;186:916–7.

45. Harmanli OH, Cheng GY, Nyirjesy P, et al. Urinary tract infections in women with bacterial vaginosis. Obstet Gynecol 2000;95:710–2.

46. Scholes D, Hooton TM, Roberts PL, et al. Risk factors associated with acute pyelonephritis in healthy women. Ann Intern Med 2005;142:20–7.

47. Dwyer LL, Harris-Kojetin LD, Valverde RH, et al. Infections in long-term care populations in the United States. J Am Geriatr Soc 2013;61:342–9.

48. Regenbogen SE, Read TE, Roberts PL, et al. Urinary tract infection after colon and rectal resections: more common than predicted by risk-adjustment models. J Am Coll Surg 2011;213:784–92.

49. Jackson D, Higgins E, Bracken J, et al. Antibiotic prophylaxis for urinary tract infection after midurethral sling: a randomized controlled trial. Female Pelvic Med Reconstr Surg 2013;19:137–41.
50. Nygaard I, Brubaker L, Chai TC, et al. Risk factors for urinary tract infection following incontinence surgery. Int Urogynecol J 2011;22:1255–65.
51. Eriksson I, Gustafson Y, Fagerstrom L, et al. Prevalence and factors associated with urinary tract infections (UTIs) in very old women. Arch Gerontol Geriatr 2010;50:132–5.
52. Caljouw MA, den Elzen WP, Cools HJ, et al. Predictive factors of urinary tract infections among the oldest old in the general population. A population-based prospective follow-up study. BMC Med 2011;9:57.
53. Hirji I, Guo Z, Andersson SW, et al. Incidence of urinary tract infection among patients with type 2 diabetes in the UK General Practice Research Database (GPRD). J Diabetes Complications 2012;26:513–6.
54. Saliba W, Barnett-Griness O, Rennert G. The association between obesity and urinary tract infection. Eur J Intern Med 2013;24:127–31.
55. Scholes D, Hawn TR, Roberts PL, et al. Family history and risk of recurrent cystitis and pyelonephritis in women. J Urol 2010;184:564–9.
56. Hawn TR, Scholes D, Wang H, et al. Genetic variation of the human urinary tract innate immune response and asymptomatic bacteriuria in women. PLoS One 2009;4:e8300.
57. Hawn TR, Scholes D, Li SS, et al. Toll-like receptor polymorphisms and susceptibility to urinary tract infections in adult women. PLoS One 2009;4:e5990.
58. Ragnarsdottir B, Svanborg C. Susceptibility to acute pyelonephritis or asymptomatic bacteriuria: host-pathogen interaction in urinary tract infections. Pediatr Nephrol 2012;27:2017–29.
59. Little P, Merriman R, Turner S, et al. Presentation, pattern, and natural course of severe symptoms, and role of antibiotics and antibiotic resistance among patients presenting with suspected uncomplicated urinary tract infection in primary care: observational study. BMJ 2010;340:b5633.
60. Foxman B. The epidemiology of urinary tract infection. Nat Rev Urol 2010;7:653–60.
61. Kim K, Lee CC, Rhee JE, et al. The effects of an institutional care map on the admission rates and medical costs in women with acute pyelonephritis. Acad Emerg Med 2008;15:319–23.
62. Jolley JA, Kim S, Wing DA. Acute pyelonephritis and associated complications during pregnancy in 2006 in US hospitals. J Matern Fetal Neonatal Med 2012;25:2494–8.
63. Al-Hasan MN, Eckel-Passow JE, Baddour LM. Bacteremia complicating gram-negative urinary tract infections: a population-based study. J Infect 2010;60:278–85.
64. Marschall J, Zhang L, Foxman B, et al. Both host and pathogen factors predispose to Escherichia coli urinary-source bacteremia in hospitalized patients. Clin Infect Dis 2012;54:1692–8.
65. Melzer M, Welch C. Outcomes in UK patients with hospital-acquired bacteraemia and the risk of catheter-associated urinary tract infections. Postgrad Med J 2013;89:329–34.

Approach to a Positive Urine Culture in a Patient Without Urinary Symptoms

Barbara W. Trautner, MD, PhD[a,b,*], Larissa Grigoryan, MD, PhD[c]

KEYWORDS

- Asymptomatic bacteriuria • Urinary tract infection • Antibacterial agents
- Guidelines implementation

KEY POINTS

- Asymptomatic bacteriuria (ASB) is defined by the presence of bacteria in an uncontaminated urine sample collected from a patient without signs or symptoms referable to the urinary tract.
- ASB is distinguished from symptomatic urinary tract infection by the absence of signs and symptoms of urinary tract infection or by determination that a nonurinary cause accounts for the patient's symptoms.
- ASB is a very common condition in diverse patient groups.
- Overtreatment of ASB with antibiotics is also very common, particularly in patients who are hospitalized, have urinary catheters, or live in a nursing home setting.
- Unnecessary antimicrobial treatment of ASB confers harm to the individual and to society.

Disclosure Statement: This work was supported by grants from the Department of Veterans Affairs [VA HSR&D IIR 09-104 and VA RRP 12-433] and the National Institutes of Health [NIH DK092293] to BW Trautner. This manuscript is the result of work supported with resources and use of facilities at the Houston VA Center for Innovations in Quality, Effectiveness and Safety [CIN13-413] at the Michael E. DeBakey VA Medical Center, Houston, TX. The opinions expressed reflect those of the authors and not necessarily those of the Department of Veterans Affairs, the US government, the NIH and Baylor College of Medicine. The NIH had no role in the design and conduct of the study; the collection, management, analysis and interpretation of the data; or the preparation, review or approval of the manuscript. L. Grigoryan's research activities were supported by National Research Service Award # 5 T32 HP10031.

[a] Department of Medicine, Center for Innovations in Quality, Effectiveness and Safety (IQuESt), Michael E. DeBakey Veterans Affairs Medical Center, 2002 Holcombe Boulevard, Houston, TX 77030, USA; [b] Section of Infectious Diseases, Department of Medicine, Baylor College of Medicine, One Baylor Plaza, Houston, TX 77030, USA; [c] Department of Family and Community Medicine, Baylor College of Medicine, 3701 Kirby, Houston, TX 77098, USA
* Corresponding author. Center for Innovations in Quality, Effectiveness and Safety (IQuESt), Michael E. DeBakey Veterans Affairs Medical Center, 2002 Holcombe Boulevard, Houston, TX 77030.
E-mail address: trautner@bcm.edu

Infect Dis Clin N Am 28 (2014) 15–31
http://dx.doi.org/10.1016/j.idc.2013.09.005
0891-5520/14/$ – see front matter Published by Elsevier Inc.

INTRODUCTION
Definition of Asymptomatic Bacteriuria

In most patient populations, interpretation of a positive urine culture depends on the presence or absence of associated symptoms. The definitions used in this review are those of the Infectious Diseases Society of America (IDSA) guidelines concerning asymptomatic bacteriuria (ASB) (2005) and catheter-associated urinary tract infection, or CAUTI (2010).[1,2] In a patient without signs and symptoms of urinary origin, the presence of bacteria in a noncontaminated urine specimen is defined as ASB.[3] In contrast, urinary tract infection (UTI) requires the presence of urinary-specific symptoms or signs in a patient who has both bacteriuria and no other identified source of infection.[1,4] The definition of ASB requires isolation of the same organism in 2 consecutive voided urine specimens for women, one voided urine specimen for men, and, in addition, from a single urine specimen collected via urinary catheter in both sexes.[2] Neither the type of bacterial species isolated from the urine nor the presence of pyuria can be used to determine whether the patient has ASB or UTI. Available evidence supports screening for and treatment of ASB in pregnant women and in patients undergoing invasive urologic procedures.[3] In most other patient groups, there is convincing evidence that neither screening nor treatment lead to improved clinical outcomes.[3] Unnecessary antibiotics given to treat ASB can cause harm in terms of antibiotic resistance, adverse drug effects, and wasted expense.[5]

These definitions are hard to apply in clinical settings, particularly in the patient populations in which ASB is most common—catheterized patients, nursing home patients, and patients in intensive care units (ICUs). The lack of specific diagnostic tests to distinguish UTI from ASB means that the diagnosis of ASB entirely depends on clinical assessment of the patient's symptoms or lack thereof. Many hospitalized or institutionalized patients may be unable to express their symptoms, and nonurinary symptoms are often attributed to bacteriuria in such patients.[6–8] Another challenge is that the diagnosis of ASB requires that the clinician ignore powerful stimuli for the use of antimicrobial agents, namely a positive urine culture result and pyuria. Other incorrect mental cues, such as reliance on urine color or urine odor, may also lead to misdiagnosis.[9] Human microbiome studies are disproving the dictum that normal bladders are sterile,[10] but the conviction that untreated bacteriuria will lead to harm persists.[11]

This review focuses on the epidemiology of ASB and its clinical significance. The review covers appropriate management of ASB in various patient populations, delineating where evidence is not adequate to support recommendations and discussing what evidence is able to guide the clinician in these areas of uncertainty. Also summarized are the growing body of published interventions that have been used to prevent overtreatment of ASB. ASB in children is not addressed, because the pathogenesis differs from that of ASB in the adult.[12] Furthermore, this review does not discuss symptomatic UTI or acute cystitis, which requires treatment with antibiotics to relieve symptoms[13] and can lead to pyelonephritis when untreated.[14] Asymptomatic funguria, management of ASB in patients undergoing urologic surgery, and management of ASB in renal transplant patients are addressed in other articles in this issue. The overall purpose of this review is to promote an awareness of ASB as a distinct condition and to empower clinicians to withhold antibiotics in situations in which antimicrobial treatment of bacteriuria is not indicated.

EPIDEMIOLOGY AND SIGNIFICANCE OF ASB
ASB is Very Common

In 2008 the Centers for Disease Control and Prevention published new surveillance definitions for CAUTI to be used by the National Healthcare Safety Network, the United

States' most widely used health care–associated infection tracking system. In keeping with the increased awareness of the distinction between UTI and ASB, ASB was excluded from urologic conditions to detect and report, in contrast to earlier definitions.[4] Presumably, the decision to exclude ASB was based on the growing awareness that ASB is not a clinically relevant condition in most populations. Changing the definition, however, was not accompanied by any change in the proportion of positive urine cultures treated with antibiotics in a large, academic medical center; such change is unlikely without an active intervention.[15] Unfortunately, the current lack of standards for detecting and reporting ASB means that published epidemiology of this condition in the United States is based on data collected before 2008[16,17] or is from smaller studies.[18,19] Before this definition change, a point prevalence study in Veterans Affairs nursing homes in 2007 found that ASB accounted for 10% of all nursing home–acquired infections, second only to UTI and skin infections.[16] National surveillance data from 1990 through 2007 showed a significant decline in ASB rates in all ICU types.[17] Estimated declines in ASB incidence ranged from 28.5% (95% CI, 20.1%–35.9%; medical/surgical without a major teaching affiliation) to 71.8% (95% CI 68.0%–75.2%; medical/surgical with a major teaching affiliation). These declines suggest that CAUTI prevention efforts in some ICUs may reduce ASB as well as CAUTI.

Risk factors for ASB include older age, female sex, and abnormalities of the genitourinary tract (**Box 1**). For example, the prevalence of ASB in healthy young women is 1% to 5%, while women older than 70 years living in the community have a risk greater than 15%.[20] Genetic factors may predispose certain women to ASB.[21] In men, a higher postvoid residual is associated with ASB, and older men are at higher risk for prostatic enlargement, which in turn creates a higher postvoid residual.[22] Whether diabetes itself creates a predisposition to ASB is not entirely clear. A single-center study in 511 diabetic and 97 nondiabetic subjects found a similar incidence of ASB in both groups.[23] However, a meta-analysis of 22 studies of ASB in diabetic versus nondiabetic subjects brought more depth to this topic. The point prevalence of

---

Box 1
Risk factors for bacteriuria in general

Sexual activity[a]

Use of diaphragm with spermicide[a]

Older age

Female sex

Diabetes mellitus

Neurogenic bladder

Hemodialysis

Urinary retention

Urinary catheter use

  Indwelling

  Intermittent

  External (condom)

[a] In sexually active, nonpregnant women ages 18–40.[28]
Data from Colgan R, Nicolle LE, McGlone A, et al. Asymptomatic bacteriuria in adults. Am Fam Physician 2006;74:985–90.

ASB was higher in both women (14.2 vs 5.1%; 2.6[1.6–4.1]) and men (2.3 vs 0.8%; 3.7 [1.3–10.2]) with diabetes than in healthy control subjects.[24]

In patients with indwelling urinary catheters, the most important risk factor for bacteriuria is the duration of catheterization.[25] Antimicrobial agents decrease the risk of bacteriuria for an initial 4 days of catheterization but are not of benefit and predispose to resistant organisms in patients catheterized longer than 4 days.[26] Because National Healthcare Safety Network surveillance for CAUTI by definition includes only patients with indwelling catheters (Foley catheters), the risk of bacteriuria with other catheter types is not well-documented. A study in 7866 inpatients on acute medicine and nursing home units over the course of 1 year documented 1009 catheter-associated, positive urine cultures. Of these, 376 (37.3%) were from external (condom) catheters, and more of the urine cultures collected from condom catheters were positive than those collected from indwelling catheters (77.1% vs 55%, respectively, P<.001).[27] Strategies to reduce CAUTI by substituting external catheters for indwelling catheters could inadvertently lead to increased antimicrobial overuse for ASB if the risk of bacteriuria with condom catheters proves to be a general phenomenon.

Clinical Outcomes Associated with ASB

Studies of the clinical impact of ASB are often confounded by the differences between persons who do and who do not have ASB at baseline. For example, 490 generally healthy women were included in a prospective study to assess the association between bacteriuria and renal function; of these, 48 had *Escherichia coli* bacteriuria at baseline. Over a mean of 12 years of follow-up, no association was found between *E coli* bacteriuria and a decline in renal function.[29] A subsequent analysis in generally the same cohort found that *E coli* bacteriuria at baseline was associated with development of hypertension, but even at baseline, the *E coli* bacteriuria group had a higher incidence of hypertension.[30]

Application of modern molecular typing techniques to samples from a prior trial of treatment versus nontreatment of ASB in diabetic women[31] offers insight on why treatment of ASB is ineffective and even potentially harmful in this population.[32] Women with diabetes and *E coli* bacteriuria were randomized to treatment for ASB (every 3 months) or no treatment. Among the 57 women in the treatment group, 76% of treatment regimens were followed by recurrent *E coli* bacteriuria, most of which (64%) involved a new strain of *E coli*. Women in the treatment group received an average of 3 courses of antimicrobial therapy, but some were treated up to 15 times. Antimicrobial treatment did not prevent recurrence but instead resulted in strain changeover. A similar phenomenon was reported in a prospective study of 330 community dwelling women ≥80 years old, followed with serial urine cultures.[33] Forty percent of women with ASB carried the same strain of *E coli* for 18 months, but antibiotic treatment led to strain turnover. Spontaneous strain turnover was also common, suggesting recolonization. In this study, the women with ASB at baseline were more likely to have symptomatic UTI over the following 24 months than those without ASB (P = .019), but the only confounding variable explicitly considered in analysis was age.

Overtreatment of ASB is Very Common

Failure to recognize ASB as a distinct condition from UTI has negative clinical consequences, namely, overuse of antibiotics. These consequences include "collateral damage" or ecological adverse effects of antibiotic use, as well as the risks of cumulative antibiotic exposure to the individual patient.[5,34,35] In 2013 the American Board of Internal Medicine identified treatment of ASB as one of the top 5 excessive health care practices in geriatrics in its "Choosing Wisely" campaign.[36] The Centers for Disease

Control and Prevention "Get Smart: Know When Antibiotics Work" campaign promotes conservative use of antibiotics, including using antibiotics to treat infection but not colonization; ASB in this context would be considered bladder colonization.[37] The cumulative impact of antimicrobial overuse on the antimicrobial susceptibility of human pathogens impairs the effectiveness of current and future antimicrobial agents.[38] In a 2-year Swedish community study, restriction of trimethoprim-containing drugs did not lead to any change in the trimethoprim resistance rate in *E coli*, thus raising the ominous concern that antimicrobial resistance may be irreversible.[39]

Unfortunately, mismanagement of ASB—or inappropriate treatment with antibiotics—is an epidemic condition.[40] Multiple studies from the United States and Canada have evaluated how often patients with ASB receive antimicrobial agents for suspected UTI (**Table 1**). All have found substantial rates of overtreatment, ranging from 20% in an emergency room study[41] to 83% in a nursing home setting.[42] Several of these studies reported high rates of overtreatment in catheterized patients, illustrating how difficult it is to interpret a positive urine culture in this population. Another concern is that many of the days of antimicrobial therapy given for ASB are unnecessary. In one study in catheterized inpatients, 201 (69%) of 293 days of antibiotic therapy to treat the urine were unnecessary.[43] A 3-year retrospective study of patients with vancomycin-resistant enterococci in their urine documented that greater than 200 days of antimicrobial therapy were not indicated, resulting in $50,000 in unnecessary antimicrobial costs.[44]

MANAGEMENT OF ASB
Patient Groups with ASB Who Should Routinely Be Treated

Current guidelines recommend ASB screening and treatment in pregnant women and patients undergoing selected urologic procedures.[2,45] A recent meta-analysis comparing antibiotics versus no treatment for pregnant women with ASB found that the treatment substantially reduced the risk of pyelonephritis.[46] The relationship between ASB, low birth weight, and preterm delivery is less well established.[47] In a *Cochrane Review*, antibiotic treatment was associated with a reduction in the incidence of low birth weight but not with preterm delivery.[46] However, poor methodological quality of studies included limits the strength of conclusions from this meta-analysis. Moreover, the definition of prematurity has changed since the 1960s, when most of these studies were conducted. Three more recent observational studies reported an increased risk of preterm birth with ASB in pregnancy.[48–50] An ongoing Dutch trial is evaluating whether nitrofurantoin treatment of low-risk, pregnant women with ASB is effective in reducing the risk of preterm delivery and/or pyelonephritis and adverse neonatal outcome.[51]

There is no consensus in the literature on screening frequency, the duration of therapy, or the choice of antibiotic for ASB in pregnancy.[47] A *Cochrane Review* of different antibiotic regimens to treat ASB in pregnancy found 5 comparative trials, 4 of which tested currently used antimicrobial agents: fosfomycin, cefuroxime, pivmecillinam, ampicillin, cephalexin, and nitrofurantoin.[52] Each trial examined a different antibiotic regimen, so no conclusions can be drawn about the most effective antibiotic regimen for ASB of pregnancy. However, in the most recent and largest of these 5 studies, a 7-day course of nitrofurantoin was shown to be more effective at achieving bacteriologic cure at 14 days posttreatment than a 1-day course of nitrofurantoin.[53] In another *Cochrane Review* on the treatment duration for ASB, the cure rate was higher for the 4- to 7-day treatment than for the 1-day treatment.[54]

Table 1
Studies documenting widespread inappropriate use of antibiotics for ASB

Reference	Country	Study Design	Study Population	Findings
Hecker et al,[88] 2003	USA	Prospective, observation over 14 d	129 inpatients	99 of 576 (17%) unnecessary days of antibiotics were for ASB
Dalen et al,[89] 2005	Canada	Prospective, observation over 26 d	29 inpatients with urinary catheters, positive urine cultures, and no symptoms of UTI	15 (52%) were prescribed unnecessary antimicrobials
Cope et al,[18] 2009	USA	Retrospective review over 3 mo	197 inpatients with urinary catheters and positive urine cultures	Of 169 treated episodes of bacteriuria, 53 (31%) were ASB
Gandhi et al,[90] 2009	USA	Retrospective review over 3 mo	414 inpatients	Of 49 patients who were treated for UTI, 13 (26%) had ASB
Silver et al,[6] 2009	Canada	Prospective, observation over 1 y	137 inpatients with positive urine cultures	43 (64%) patients with ASB were treated
Khawcharoenporn et al,[41] 2011	USA	Retrospective review over 8 mo	676 emergency department patients with positive urine cultures	37 (20%) of 184 patients with ASB were treated with antibiotics
Werner et al,[86] 2011	USA	Prospective, observation over 6 wk	226 inpatients who received fluoroquinolones	Of 690 d of unnecessary fluoroquinolone therapy, 158 (23%) were for ASB
Lin et al,[19] 2012	USA	Retrospective review over 3 mo	339 inpatients, outpatients and emergency department patients with enterococcal bacteriuria	60 (32.8%) of 183 episodes of ASB inappropriately treated with antibiotics
Phillips et al,[42] 2012	USA	Retrospective review over 6 mo	16 catheterized nursing home patients	19 (83%) of 23 treated episodes were asymptomatic
Chiu et al,[43] 2013	Canada	Retrospective review over 6 mo	80 inpatients with indwelling urinary catheters	23 (58%) of 40 patients with a positive culture result were prescribed unnecessary antimicrobials
D'Agata et al,[60] 2013	USA	Prospective over 12 mo	72 nursing home residents with dementia	82 (75%) of 110 episodes of suspected UTI were prescribed unnecessary antibiotics
Heintz et al,[44] 2013	USA	Retrospective review over 3 y	252 patients with vancomycin-resistant enterococci in urine	33 (21.3%) of 155 asymptomatic patients were treated

Patient Groups with ASB Who Should Not Be Treated

- Non-pregnant women
- Diabetic women
- Elderly persons living in the community
- Persons with spinal cord injury
- Catheterized patients while the catheter remains in place

Several prospective studies had established that ASB in premenopausal, nonpregnant women is not associated with long-term adverse outcomes and treatment of ASB neither decreases the frequency of symptomatic infection nor prevents further episodes of ASB.[2] More recently, a randomized, non-placebo-controlled trial studied ASB specifically in women with recurrent UTI. This study enrolled 673 women ages 18 to 40 with recurrent UTI and ASB at baseline.[55] Women were split into 2 groups, treated with a single course of antibiotics or not treated, and followed for 12 months. At the last follow-up, 41 (13.1%) in the untreated group and 169 (46.8%) in the treated group had a symptomatic UTI (RR, 3.17; 95% CI, 2.55–3.90; $P<.0001$). This finding is in line with a prior observational cohort study that reported women who had received antimicrobials during the previous 15 to 28 days were at higher risk for UTI.[56] A plausible explanation is that antibiotics may predispose to UTI by altering the flora colonizing the vagina.

Randomized, controlled trials of ASB screening and/or treatment have established the lack of efficacy in diabetic women, patients with spinal cord injury, catheterized patients, and older adults.[2] In randomized, controlled trials including patients with spinal cord injury, rates of symptomatic urinary infection and recurrence of bacteriuria were similar in patients receiving antibiotics and those who did not.[57,58] Antibiotic treatment in catheterized patients did not decrease symptomatic episodes and increased emergence of more resistant organisms.[2]

Patient Groups in Which ASB is Particularly Hard to Diagnose

Nursing home patients

Clinical trials in elderly nursing home residents have consistently found no benefits with treatment of ASB.[45] The minimum clinical criteria to initiate antimicrobial therapy in the general nursing home population were established in 2001.[59] Despite extensive research demonstrating a lack of benefit and a potential for harm for antibiotic use for ASB, nursing home residents frequently receive an antibiotic for ASB. In a recent study investigating antibiotic use among residents in 4 nursing homes, half of the antibiotic prescriptions were for residents with no documented UTI symptoms.[42] In another study, only 11% of suspected UTI episodes in nursing home residents with advanced dementia had both the symptoms and the laboratory criteria necessary for diagnosis of UTI; 82 (75%) of the 110 episodes that did not meet the minimum criteria for treatment were treated with antimicrobials.[60] The usefulness of urinary specimens in diagnosing UTI was questionable, because the proportion of episodes with a positive urinalysis and culture was similar for those that met (83%) and did not meet (78%) minimum clinical criteria ($P = .06$).[60]

ICU patients

ICU patients and older institutionalized patients have in common a limited ability to communicate. Most patients who are hospitalized in ICUs receive an indwelling urinary catheter to monitor urine output; many are also on ventilators and have centrally placed vascular catheters. Thus, determining the source of fever in an ICU patient with an indwelling catheter is particularly difficult, particularly as catheter-associated bacteriuria is so common. A study in a French ICU of 2 different urinary catheter types found that 9.6% of patients developed bacteriuria on day 12 ± 7, although these study catheters had been placed under ideal conditions.[61] In a trauma ICU study in 510 patients, the tendency to blame fever on bacteriuria was not supported by evidence. Although there was a significant association between having a urine culture and having a fever (P<.001), bacteriuria was not associated with fever, leukocytosis, or the combination of fever and leukocytosis.[62] A systematic review and meta-analysis of 11 studies in adult ICU patients with catheter-associated bacteriuria (with or without symptoms of CAUTI) found that bacteriuria was associated with increased mortality in unadjusted analysis. However, after restricting the analysis to studies that adjusted for other outcome predictors, bacteriuria was no longer associated with mortality but was possibly related to a small increase in length of stay (mean difference +2.6 days; 95% CI 2.3–3.0).[63] This finding is in accord with the results of a randomized clinical trial in 60 patients in ICUs who were asymptomatic and catheterized with positive urine cultures.[64] Treatment of the bacteriuria with antibiotics and catheter exchange did not reduce the rate of urosepsis, bacteremia, or positive urine cultures on day 15 after enrollment.

Patient Groups with ASB and Inadequate Evidence to Guide Management

Evidence to guide management of preoperative ASB before nonurologic procedures is limited. A recent study addressed whether preoperative screening for and treatment of ASB in patients undergoing cardiovascular, orthopedic, or vascular procedures confers benefits.[65] Among patients with a preoperative culture, patients with bacteriuria and those without bacteriuria were compared for postoperative complications. Surgical site infection was similarly frequent among patients with bacteriuria versus those without, whereas postoperative UTI was more frequent among patients with bacteriuria (9% vs 2%, P = .01). Among the 54 patients with a positive screening culture, a greater proportion of treated patients developed a surgical site infection compared with untreated patients (45% vs 14%, P = .03). However, the findings from this small observational study should be interpreted with caution because of the high likelihood of confounding factors.

Few studies have evaluated the impact of bacteriuria in patients undergoing major joint replacement surgery.[66] Most of these studies had retrospective design and were published over a decade ago.[66] In one prospective study of hip and knee arthroplasty, preoperative bacteriuria was not associated with subsequent joint infection at 1 year after the procedure.[67] However, all patients in this study had received preoperative cefuroxime therapy. In a recent prospective randomized study including 471 patients, ASB occurred in 8 (3.5%) of 228 patients undergoing total hip arthroplasty and in 38 (15.6%) of 243 patients undergoing hemiarthroplasty.[68] Patients were randomized to receive specific antibiotic treatment or no treatment. No case of prosthetic joint infection from urinary origin was identified in any study group in this trial. However, the sample size might have been too small to detect an effect in this trial. Whether screening for and treating bacteriuria before prosthetic joint implantation confers any clinical benefit is unknown.

Another area lacking definitive evidence in the IDSA guidelines is in how to manage existing bacteriuria at the time of removal of a urinary catheter. Since publication of the guidelines, additional literature on this topic provided enough data to perform a meta-analysis.[69–71] In a systematic review and meta-analysis of pooled data from 7 studies, antibiotic prophylaxis was beneficial with an absolute reduction in risk symptomatic UTI of 5.8% between intervention and control groups and a risk ratio of 0.45 (95% 0.28–0.72).[72] One obvious practical consideration is that to implement this approach,

Table 2
Interventional studies to decrease ASB overtreatment

Reference	Study Setting	Study Design	Intervention	Outcomes
Loeb et al,[73] 2005	Nursing homes	Cluster randomized controlled trial	Multifaceted, algorithm use taught by case scenarios in interactive sessions	Fewer courses of antimicrobials for suspected UTI in intervention homes (1.17/1000 resident days) than in control homes (1.59/1000 resident days)
Bonnal et al,[74] 2008	University-affiliated geriatric hospital	Audit before and after intervention	Pocket card plus post-prescription audit and feedback for positive urine cultures managed inappropriately	Antibiotic use for ASB decreased from 196 d during the preintervention year to 150 d during the intervention year, $P = .007$
Zabarsky et al,[77] 2008	Veterans Affairs long-term care facility	Audit before and after intervention	Pocket cards, educational sessions, audit, and feedback	Decrease in urine cultures sent, reduction in treatment of ASB and in total days of antimicrobial therapy (from 168 to 117 per 1000 patient-days, $P<.001$)
Pavese et al,[78] 2009	University-affiliated hospital	Controlled audit before and after intervention	Distribution of guidelines and report plus a 1 h interactive educational session	Antibiotic use for ASB in intervention group decreased from 74% before intervention to 17% afterward ($P = .01$)
Linares et al,[79] 2011	Veterans Affairs hospital	Audit before and after intervention	Memorandum placed in electronic medical record if antibiotics were inappropriate	Mean duration of treatment of ASB decreased from 6.3 d in control group to 2.2 d in intervention group ($P<.001$)
Egger et al,[75] 2013	Teaching hospital	Before and after	Multifaceted, implementation of guidelines, catheter reminders, and Internet-based teaching cases	ASB treatment dropped significantly from 22 to 10 treatment days per 1000 patient days (incidence rate ratio 0.46, 95% CI 0.33–0.63)
Pettersson et al,[76] 2011	Nursing homes	Cluster randomized controlled trial	Education about UTI with feedback on baseline antibiotic prescription data	The proportion of overall infections treated with an antibiotic decreased significantly by −0.124 (95% CI −0.228, −0.019) compared with the control group

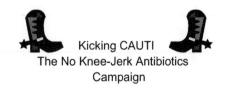

Kicking CAUTI
The No Knee-Jerk Antibiotics
Campaign

Catheter-Associated UTI (CAUTI) vs Asymptomatic Bacteriuria

(Patient with urinary catheter or catheter use within 48 hours)

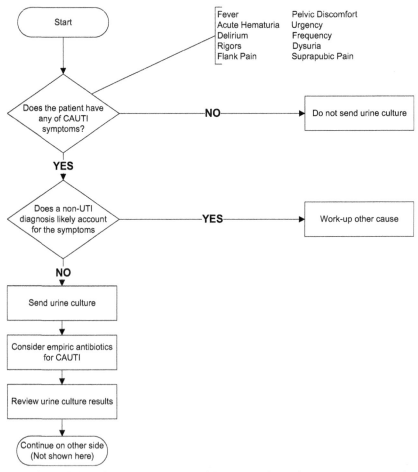

Fig. 1. Validated algorithm to assist in clinical decision-making about positive urine cultures in catheterized patients. The focus of the algorithm is on reminding the clinician to stop and think about 2 key questions before reflexively prescribing antibiotics for bacteriuria. (*From* Trautner BW, Bhimani RD, Amspoker AB, et al. Development and validation of an algorithm to recalibrate mental models and reduce diagnostic errors associated with catheter-associated bacteriuria. BMC Med Inform Decis Mak 2013;13:48.)

testing of urine before catheter removal would need to be performed in time to have urine culture results at catheter removal or shortly thereafter.

Prevention of Inappropriate Treatment of ASB

Several interventional studies have addressed the issue of inappropriate treatment of ASB (**Table 2**).[73–79] These guidelines implementation interventions were heterogeneous and measured different outcomes. However, all strategies went beyond passive education, many incorporating audit and feedback or interactive learning, and all reported a decrease in antibiotic use. One common theme of these diverse and successful strategies is that they engendered medical mindfulness, or made a thoughtful clinical decision, rather than reflexive use of antibiotics.[80,81] Our ongoing intervention, entitled "Kicking CAUTI: the No Knee-Jerk Antibiotics Campaign," encourages clinicians to stop and think before ordering cultures and prescribing antibiotics for catheter-associated bacteriuria.[82] The 2 main tools used in the intervention are (1) an evidence-based, actionable algorithm that distills the guidelines into a streamlined clinical pathway and encourages a mindful pause (**Fig. 1**),[9] and (2) case-based audit and feedback to train clinicians to use the algorithm. This algorithm was developed with input from the authors of the IDSA ASB and CAUTI guidelines, and use of this algorithm improved nonexperts' diagnostic accuracy of ASB versus CAUTI when applied retrospectively to actual cases.[9] Overall, these interventional studies offer hope that guidelines implementation can decrease antimicrobial overuse for ASB. The design of interventions to reduce overutilization for ASB should integrate behavioral theory so that the underlying cognitive, behavioral, and financial drivers are addressed.[83] Interventions should be tailored to fit specific goals and also should address the root causes of inappropriate prescribing.[84]

SUMMARY

The most important and far-reaching consequences of ASB are not the impact of this condition per se on the individual patient but the negative consequences of overtreatment of ASB in terms of antimicrobial resistance, suprainfections, and unnecessary costs. Increasing awareness that ASB usually does not require treatment led to eliminating ASB from infection control surveillance programs, but this change in surveillance definitions will not in itself change clinical practice.[85] Likewise, although the epidemic of overtreatment of ASB has been thoroughly documented, these descriptions in themselves will not lead to a solution unless their data serve as a foundation for interventions to optimize management of ASB. Unfortunately, awareness that overtreatment of ASB is a problem has preceded any immediate widespread solutions; currently many of the episodes diagnosed and treated as CAUTI in the hospital are really ASB.[19,43,86] In the future, perhaps some of the resources that have been channeled into reducing CAUTI and other health care–associated infections[87] can be used to support effective ASB guidelines implementation programs.

REVIEW CRITERIA

A search strategy was developed that covers the main subject area of the review (ASB) and a systematic literature search in the Medline database was performed. The search was limited to articles published in English between 2002 and 2013. The search initially used the following search strategy: "Asymptomatic bacteriuria AND (anti-bacterial agents OR antimicrobial OR antimicrobials OR anti-microbial OR anti-microbials OR antibiotic OR antibiotics OR anti-bacterial OR antibacterial OR antibacterials)."

The following abstract appraisal criteria were used:

- Title or abstract addresses one or more of the study questions
- Title or abstract identifies primary research or systematically conducted secondary research

Reference lists of retrieved articles (particularly older literature) and abstracts from key journals were also hand-searched. Additional search strategies were used for each subtopic, including the following search terms, "catheter-associated urinary tract infection," "bacteriuria and diabetes," "bacteriuria and non-pregnant," "bacteriuria and spinal cord injury," "bacteriuria and intensive care OR ICU OR critically ill," "bacteriuria in elderly," "bacteriuria and nursing home," "antibiotic overuse," "performance measures," "*Escherichia coli* and bacteriuria," "bacteriuria and pregnancy," "bacteriuria and preoperative," "bacteriuria and urinary catheter removal," "*Escherichia coli*," and "bacteriuria and anti-bacterial agents," among others.

REFERENCES

1. Hooton TM, Bradley SF, Cardenas DD, et al. Diagnosis, prevention, and treatment of catheter-associated urinary tract infection in adults: 2009 International Clinical Practice Guidelines from the Infectious Diseases Society of America. Clin Infect Dis 2010;50:625–63.
2. Nicolle LE, Bradley S, Colgan R, et al. Infectious Diseases Society of America guidelines for the diagnosis and treatment of asymptomatic bacteriuria in adults. Clin Infect Dis 2005;40:643–54.
3. Lin K, Fajardo K. Screening for asymptomatic bacteriuria in adults: evidence for the U.S. preventive services task force reaffirmation recommendation statement. Ann Intern Med 2008;149:W20–4.
4. Horan TC, Andrus M, Dudeck M. CDC/NHSN surveillance definition of healthcare-associated infection and criteria for specific types of infections in the acute care setting. Am J Infect Control 2008;36(5):309–32.
5. Gupta K, Hooton TM, Naber KG, et al. International Clinical Practice Guidelines for the treatment of acute uncomplicated cystitis and pyelonephritis in women: a 2010 update by the Infectious Diseases Society of America and the European Society for Microbiology and Infectious Diseases. Clin Infect Dis 2011;52:e103–20.
6. Silver SA, Baillie L, Simor AE. Positive urine cultures: a major cause of inappropriate antimicrobial use in hospitals? Can J Infect Dis Med Microbiol 2009;20:107–11.
7. Walker S, McGeer A, Simor AE, et al. Why are antibiotics prescribed for asymptomatic bacteriuria in institutionalized elderly people? A qualitative study of physicians' and nurses' perceptions. CMAJ 2000;163:273–7.
8. Drinka PJ, Crnich CJ. Diagnostic accuracy of criteria for urinary tract infection in a cohort of nursing home residents. J Am Geriatr Soc 2008;56:376–7 [author reply: 378].
9. Trautner BW, Bhimani RD, Amspoker AB, et al. Development and validation of an algorithm to recalibrate mental models and reduce diagnostic errors associated with catheter-associated bacteriuria. BMC Med Inform Decis Mak 2013;13:48.
10. Fouts DE, Pieper R, Szpakowski S, et al. Integrated next-generation sequencing of 16S rDNA and metaproteomics differentiate the healthy urine microbiome from asymptomatic bacteriuria in neuropathic bladder associated with spinal cord injury. J Transl Med 2012;10:174.

11. Drekonja DM, Abbo LM, Kuskowski MA, et al. A survey of resident physicians' knowledge regarding urine testing and subsequent antimicrobial treatment. Am J Infect Control 2013;41(10):892–6.
12. Montini G, Tullus K, Hewitt I. Febrile urinary tract infections in children. N Engl J Med 2011;365:239–50.
13. Little P, Moore MV, Turner S, et al. Effectiveness of five different approaches in management of urinary tract infection: randomised controlled trial. BMJ 2010; 340:c199.
14. Falagas ME, Kotsantis IK, Vouloumanou EK, et al. Antibiotics versus placebo in the treatment of women with uncomplicated cystitis: a meta-analysis of randomized controlled trials. J Infect 2009;58:91–102.
15. Press MJ, Metlay JP. Catheter-associated urinary tract infection: does changing the definition change quality? Infect Control Hosp Epidemiol 2013;34:313–5.
16. Tsan L, Landberg R, Davis C, et al. Nursing home-associated infections in Department of Veterans Affairs community living centers. Am J Infect Control 2010;38:461–6.
17. Burton DC, Edwards JR, Srinivasan A, et al. Trends in catheter-associated urinary tract infections in adult intensive care units-United States, 1990-2007. Infect Control Hosp Epidemiol 2011;32:748–56.
18. Cope M, Cevallos ME, Cadle RM, et al. Inappropriate treatment of catheter-associated asymptomatic bacteriuria in a tertiary care hospital. Clin Infect Dis 2009;48:1182–8.
19. Lin E, Bhusal Y, Horwitz D, et al. Overtreatment of enterococcal bacteriuria. Arch Intern Med 2012;172:33–8.
20. Colgan R, Nicolle LE, McGlone A, et al. Asymptomatic bacteriuria in adults. Am Fam Physician 2006;74:985–90.
21. Hawn TR, Scholes D, Wang H, et al. Genetic variation of the human urinary tract innate immune response and asymptomatic bacteriuria in women. PLoS One 2009;4:e8300.
22. Truzzi JC, Almeida FM, Nunes EC, et al. Residual urinary volume and urinary tract infection–when are they linked? J Urol 2008;180:182–5.
23. Matteucci E, Troilo A, Leonetti P, et al. Significant bacteriuria in outpatient diabetic and non-diabetic persons. Diabet Med 2007;24:1455–9.
24. Renko M, Tapanainen P, Tossavainen P, et al. Meta-analysis of the significance of asymptomatic bacteriuria in diabetes. Diabetes Care 2011;34:230–5.
25. Shuman EK, Chenoweth CE. Recognition and prevention of healthcare-associated urinary tract infections in the intensive care unit. Crit Care Med 2010;38:S373–9.
26. Garibaldi RA, Burke JP, Dickman ML, et al. Factors predisposing to bacteriuria during indwelling urethral catheterization. N Engl J Med 1974;291:215–9.
27. Trautner BW, Patterson JE, Petersen NJ, et al. Quality gaps in documenting urinary catheter use and infectious outcomes. Infect Control Hosp Epidemiol 2013; 34:793–9.
28. Hooton TM, Scholes D, Stapleton AE, et al. A prospective study of asymptomatic bacteriuria in sexually active young women. N Engl J Med 2000;343:992–7.
29. Meiland R, Stolk RP, Geerlings SE, et al. Association between Escherichia coli bacteriuria and renal function in women: long-term follow-up. Arch Intern Med 2007;167:253–7.
30. Meiland R, Geerlings SE, Stolk RP, et al. Escherichia coli bacteriuria in female adults is associated with the development of hypertension. Int J Infect Dis 2010;14:e304–7.

31. Harding G, Zhanel G, Nicolle L, et al. Antimicrobial treatment in diabetic women with asymptomatic bacteriuria. N Engl J Med 2002;347:1576–83.

32. Dalal S, Nicolle L, Marrs CF, et al. Long-term Escherichia coli asymptomatic bacteriuria among women with diabetes mellitus. Clin Infect Dis 2009;49:491–7.

33. Rodhe N, Löfgren S, Matussek A, et al. Asymptomatic bacteriuria in the elderly: high prevalence and high turnover of strains. Scand J Infect Dis 2008;40:804–10.

34. Paterson DL. "Collateral damage" from cephalosporin or quinolone antibiotic therapy. Clin Infect Dis 2004;38(Suppl 4):S341–5.

35. Stevens V, Dumyati G, Fine LS, et al. Cumulative antibiotic exposures over time and the risk of Clostridium difficile infection. Clin Infect Dis 2011;53:42–8.

36. ABIM Foundation. Choosing Wisely: An initiative of the ABIM foundation. 2013. Available at: http://www.choosingwisely.org/doctor-patient-lists/american-geriatrics-society/. Accessed October 8, 2013.

37. Centers for Disease Control and Prevention. Get Smart: Know When Antibiotics Work. Available at: http://www.cdc.gov/getsmart/. Accessed October 8, 2013.

38. Spellberg B, Guidos R, Gilbert D, et al. The epidemic of antibiotic-resistant infections: a call to action for the medical community from the Infectious Diseases Society of America. Clin Infect Dis 2008;46:155–64.

39. Sundqvist M, Geli P, Andersson DI, et al. Little evidence for reversibility of trimethoprim resistance after a drastic reduction in trimethoprim use. J Antimicrob Chemother 2010;65:350–60.

40. Gross PA, Patel B. Reducing antibiotic overuse: a call for a national performance measure for not treating asymptomatic bacteriuria. Clin Infect Dis 2007;45:1335–7.

41. Khawcharoenporn T, Vasoo S, Ward E, et al. Abnormal urinalysis finding triggered antibiotic prescription for asymptomatic bacteriuria in the ED. Am J Emerg Med 2011;29(7):828–30.

42. Phillips CD, Adepoju O, Stone N, et al. Asymptomatic bacteriuria, antibiotic use, and suspected urinary tract infections in four nursing homes. BMC Geriatr 2012; 12:73.

43. Chiu J, Thompson GW, Austin TW, et al. Antibiotic prescribing practices for catheter urine culture results. Can J Hosp Pharm 2013;66:13–20.

44. Heintz BH, Cho S, Fujioka A, et al. Evaluation of the treatment of vancomycin-resistant enterococcal urinary tract infections in a large academic medical center. Ann Pharmacother 2013;47:159–69.

45. Nicolle LE. Asymptomatic bacteriuria: review and discussion of the IDSA guidelines. Int J Antimicrob Agents 2006;28(Suppl 1):S42–8.

46. Smaill F, Vazquez JC. Antibiotics for asymptomatic bacteriuria in pregnancy. Cochrane Database Syst Rev 2007;(2):CD000490.

47. Schnarr J, Smaill F. Asymptomatic bacteriuria and symptomatic urinary tract infections in pregnancy. Eur J Clin Invest 2008;38(Suppl 2):50–7.

48. Sheiner E, Mazor-Drey E, Levy A. Asymptomatic bacteriuria during pregnancy. J Matern Fetal Neonatal Med 2009;22:423–7.

49. Marahatta R, Dhungel BA, Pradhan P, et al. Asymptomatic bacteriurea among pregnant women visiting Nepal Medical College Teaching Hospital, Kathmandu, Nepal. Nepal Med Coll J 2011;13:107–10.

50. Ullah MA, Barman A, Siddique MA, et al. Prevalence of asymptomatic bacteriuria and its consequences in pregnancy in a rural community of Bangladesh. Bangladesh Med Res Counc Bull 2007;33:60–4.

51. Kazemier BM, Schneerberger C, De Miranda E, et al. Costs and effects of screening and treating low risk women with a singleton pregnancy for asymptomatic bacteriuria, the ASB study. BMC Pregnancy Childbirth 2012;12:52.

52. Guinto VT, De Guia B, Festin MR, et al. Different antibiotic regimens for treating asymptomatic bacteriuria in pregnancy. Cochrane Database Syst Rev 2010;(9):CD007855.
53. Lumbiganon P, Villar J, Laopaiboon M, et al. One-day compared with 7-day nitrofurantoin for asymptomatic bacteriuria in pregnancy: a randomized controlled trial. Obstet Gynecol 2009;113:339–45.
54. Widmer M, Gulmezoglu AM, Mignini L, et al. Duration of treatment for asymptomatic bacteriuria during pregnancy. Cochrane Database Syst Rev 2011;(12):CD000491.
55. Cai T, Mazzoli S, Mondaini N, et al. The role of asymptomatic bacteriuria in young women with recurrent urinary tract infections: to treat or not to treat? Clin Infect Dis 2012;55:771–7.
56. Smith HS, Hughes JP, Hooton TM, et al. Antecedent antimicrobial use increases the risk of uncomplicated cystitis in young women. Clin Infect Dis 1997;25:63–8.
57. Mohler JL, Cowen DL, Flanigan RC. Suppression and treatment of urinary tract infection in patients with an intermittently catheterized neurogenic bladder. J Urol 1987;138:336–40.
58. Maynard FM, Diokno AC. Urinary infection and complications during clean intermittent catheterization following spinal cord injury. J Urol 1984;132:943–6.
59. Loeb M, Bentley DW, Bradley S, et al. Development of minimum criteria for the initiation of antibiotics in residents of long-term-care facilities: results of a consensus conference. Infect Control Hosp Epidemiol 2001;22:120–4.
60. D'Agata E, Loeb MB, Mitchell SL. Challenges in assessing nursing home residents with advanced dementia for suspected urinary tract infections. J Am Geriatr Soc 2013;61:62–6.
61. Leone M, Albanese J, Garnier F, et al. Risk factors of nosocomial catheter-associated urinary tract infection in a polyvalent intensive care unit. Intensive Care Med 2003;29:1077–80.
62. Golob JF Jr, Claridge JA, Sando MJ, et al. Fever and leukocytosis in critically ill trauma patients: it's not the urine. Surg Infect (Larchmt) 2008;9:49–56.
63. Chant C, Smith OM, Marshall JC, et al. Relationship of catheter-associated urinary tract infection to mortality and length of stay in critically ill patients: a systematic review and meta-analysis of observational studies. Crit Care Med 2011; 39:1167–73.
64. Leone M, Perrin AS, Granier I, et al. A randomized trial of catheter change and short course of antibiotics for asymptomatic bacteriuria in catheterized ICU patients. Intensive Care Med 2007;33:726–9.
65. Drekonja DM, Zarmbinski B, Johnson JR. Preoperative urine cultures at a Veterans Affairs Medical Center. Arch Intern Med 2012;173(1):61–2.
66. Rajamanickam A, Noor S, Usmani A. Should an asymptomatic patient with an abnormal urinalysis (bacteriuria or pyuria) be treated with antibiotics prior to major joint replacement surgery? Cleve Clin J Med 2007;74(Suppl 1):S17–8.
67. Wymenga AB, van Horn JR, Theeuwes A, et al. Perioperative factors associated with septic arthritis after arthroplasty. Prospective multicenter study of 362 knee and 2,651 hip operations. Acta Orthop Scand 1992;63:665–71.
68. Cordero-Ampuero J, Gonzalez-Fernandez E, Martinez-Velez D, et al. Are antibiotics necessary in hip arthroplasty with asymptomatic bacteriuria? Seeding risk with/without treatment. Clin Orthop Relat Res 2013. [Epub ahead of print].
69. van Hees BC, Vijverberg PL, Hoorntje LE, et al. Single-dose antibiotic prophylaxis for urinary catheter removal does not reduce the risk of urinary tract

infection in surgical patients: a randomized double-blind placebo-controlled trial. Clin Microbiol Infect 2011;17:1091–4.

70. Pinochet R, Nogueira L, Cronin AM, et al. Role of short-term antibiotic therapy at the moment of catheter removal after laparoscopic radical prostatectomy. Urol Int 2010;85:415–20.

71. Pfefferkorn U, Lea S, Moldenhauer J, et al. Antibiotic prophylaxis at urinary catheter removal prevents urinary tract infections: a prospective randomized trial. Ann Surg 2009;249:573–5.

72. Marschall J, Carpenter CR, Fowler S, et al, CDC Prevention Epicenters Program. Antibiotic prophylaxis for urinary tract infections after removal of urinary catheter: meta-analysis. BMJ 2013;346:f3147.

73. Loeb M, Brazil K, Lohfeld L, et al. Effect of a multifaceted intervention on number of antimicrobial prescriptions for suspected urinary tract infections in residents of nursing homes: cluster randomised controlled trial. BMJ 2005;331:669.

74. Bonnal C, Baune B, Mion M, et al. Bacteriuria in a geriatric hospital: impact of an antibiotic improvement program. J Am Med Dir Assoc 2008;9:605–9.

75. Egger M, Balmer F, Friedli-Wuthrich H, et al. Reduction of urinary catheter use and prescription of antibiotics for asymptomatic bacteriuria in hospitalised patients in internal medicine: before-and-after intervention study. Swiss Med Wkly 2013;143:w13796.

76. Pettersson E, Vernby A, Molstad S, et al. Can a multifaceted educational intervention targeting both nurses and physicians change the prescribing of antibiotics to nursing home residents? A cluster randomized controlled trial. J Antimicrob Chemother 2011;66:2659–66.

77. Zabarsky TF, Sethi AK, Donskey CJ. Sustained reduction in inappropriate treatment of asymptomatic bacteriuria in a long-term care facility through an educational intervention. Am J Infect Control 2008;36:476–80.

78. Pavese P, Saurel N, Labarere J, et al. Does an educational session with an infectious diseases physician reduce the use of inappropriate antibiotic therapy for inpatients with positive urine culture results? A controlled before-and-after study. Infect Control Hosp Epidemiol 2009;30:596–9.

79. Linares LA, Thornton DJ, Strymish J, et al. Electronic memorandum decreases unnecessary antimicrobial use for asymptomatic bacteriuria and culture-negative pyuria. Infect Control Hosp Epidemiol 2011;32:644–8.

80. Epstein RM. Mindful practice. JAMA 1999;282:833–9.

81. Flanders SA, Saint S. Enhancing the safety of hospitalized patients: who is minding the antimicrobials? Arch Intern Med 2012;172:38–40.

82. Trautner BW, Kelly PA, Petersen N, et al. A hospital-site controlled intervention using audit and feedback to implement guidelines concerning inappropriate treatment of catheter-associated asymptomatic bacteriuria. Implement Sci 2011;6:41.

83. Naik AD, Hinojosa-Lindsey M, Arney J, et al. Choosing wisely and the perceived drivers of endoscopy use. Clin Gastroenterol Hepatol 2013;11:753–5.

84. Hulscher ME, van der Meer JW, Grol RP. Antibiotic use: how to improve it? Int J Med Microbiol 2010;300:351–6.

85. Cabana MD, Rand CS, Powe NR, et al. Why don't physicians follow clinical practice guidelines? A framework for improvement. JAMA 1999;282:1458–65.

86. Werner NL, Hecker MT, Sethi AK, et al. Unnecessary use of fluoroquinolone antibiotics in hospitalized patients. BMC Infect Dis 2011;11:187.

87. Saint S, Meddings JA, Calfee D, et al. Catheter-associated urinary tract infection and the Medicare rule changes. Ann Intern Med 2009;150:877–84.

88. Hecker MT, Aron DC, Patel NP, et al. Unnecessary use of antimicrobials in hospitalized patients: current patterns of misuse with an emphasis on the antianaerobic spectrum of activity. Arch Intern Med 2003;163:972–8.
89. Dalen DM, Zvonar RK, Jessamine PG. An evaluation of the management of asymptomatic catheter-associated bacteriuria and candiduria at The Ottawa Hospital. Can J Infect Dis Med Microbiol 2005;16:166–70.
90. Gandhi T, Flanders SA, Markovitz E, et al. Importance of urinary tract infection to antibiotic use among hospitalized patients. Infect Control Hosp Epidemiol 2009;30:193–5.

Diagnosis and Management of Urinary Tract Infection in the Emergency Department and Outpatient Settings

Sukhjit S. Takhar, MD[a], Gregory J. Moran, MD[b],*

KEYWORDS

- Cystitis • Pyelonephritis • Emergency department • Sepsis • Urolithiasis

KEY POINTS

- The extent of diagnostic work-up in emergency departments (EDs) varies widely depending on severity of illness and underlying comorbidities.
- Most patients with pyelonephritis can be successfully managed as outpatients, even if they appear seriously ill on initial presentation.
- It is important to follow-up on pending culture and susceptibility results for patients discharged home from an ED.
- Urinary obstruction should be ruled out in patients with a urinary tract infections (UTIs) and severe sepsis/septic shock. Bedside ultrasound is often used for this in an ED.

INTRODUCTION

Urinary tract infections (UTI) are common clinical conditions seen EDs. Patients with UTIs often become acutely symptomatic and seek care in an ED during off-hours, when they cannot get a timely appointment with their primary care physician, or when they do not have access to primary care. Patients who present to an ED are often more ill than those who present to an office-based practice.

Infectious disease specialists typically become involved in management of UTIs only in unusual or complicated cases (**Box 1**). In contrast, emergency physicians see a wide spectrum of illness severity, from uncomplicated cystitis to septic shock. The challenges of managing UTIs in EDs include limited history, lack of longitudinal follow-up, and lack of culture and susceptibility results. EDs frequently provide

Disclosures: Dr Takhar: None; Dr Moran has received speaking honoraria from Forest and Merck and has received clinical research funding from Astra-Zeneca and Cerexa.
[a] Department of Emergency Medicine, Brigham and Women's Hospital, Harvard Medical School, 75 Francis Street, Boston, MA 02115, USA; [b] Division of Infectious Diseases, Department of Emergency Medicine, Olive View-UCLA Medical Center, Geffen School of Medicine at UCLA, 14445 Olive View Dr., Sylmar, CA 91342, USA
* Corresponding author.
E-mail address: gmoran@ucla.edu

Infect Dis Clin N Am 28 (2014) 33–48
http://dx.doi.org/10.1016/j.idc.2013.10.003
0891-5520/14/$ – see front matter © 2014 Elsevier Inc. All rights reserved.

id.theclinics.com

Box 1
Selected characteristics that make urinary tract infections complicated

Pregnancy

Male gender

Moderate to severe diabetes or other immunosupressed state

Structural abnormalities of urinary tract (kidney stones, renal and perinephric abscess, emphysematous pyelonephritis, or polycystic kidney disease)

Functional abnormality of urinary tract (vesico-ureteral reflux, spinal cord injury, neurogenic bladder)

Hospital-acquired infections

Presence of external catheters (urethral, suprapubic, or nephrostomy tubes)

---

medical care for patients without medical insurance in the United States, and many patients have no other access to care or follow-up.

The role of the emergency physician is to determine complicated versus uncomplicated infection, make disposition decisions regarding hospitalization and level of care, and choose appropriate empiric antimicrobial treatment based on the likely bacterial etiologies and the ever-changing patterns of antimicrobial resistance. Because UTIs are common, it is also important to consider cost issues in the diagnostic evaluation and management. It may be neither practical nor advisable to send cultures for every case of uncomplicated cystitis. This article reviews the diagnostic approach to and treatment of adults presenting to EDs with UTI.

CLASSIFICATION/DEFINITIONS

UTIs can be described by their location and the presence of functional or structural abnormalities. Acute cystitis is an infection of the bladder and is referred to as a lower UTI. Pyelonephritis, an upper UTI, is more severe and can occur in conjunction with acute cystitis. In practice, it is sometimes difficult to make a clear distinction between these clinical syndromes during an ED evaluation. Uncomplicated UTIs are episodes of acute cystitis or pyelonephritis occurring in healthy premenopausal women who are not pregnant with no history of structural abnormalities or without any functional abnormalities in the urinary tract.[1–3] These infections are generally considered at lower risk for drug-resistant organisms and treatment failure. All other cases are classified as complicated infections.

Complicated UTIs are heterogeneous: broadly defined, they are associated with a condition that increases the risk of acquiring infections or failing therapy.[1,4] Distinguishing between complicated and uncomplicated is important because it influences the initial evaluation and the choice and duration of antibiotics.

EPIDEMIOLOGY

UTIs are common, with approximately half of all women reporting having at least one infection. In 2010, there were more than 3 million ED visits with a primary diagnosis of a UTI.[5,6] Of these, 84.5% were women and approximately half of all UTI presentations to an ED were among patients aged 18 to 44. Overall, the acuity of presentations to EDs is higher than those seen by primary care providers. More than 400,000 (13%) ED visits for UTIs in 2010 were for pyelonephritis, approximately 13 visits per 10,000 people. In the general population, pyelonephritis occurs in 1 case per 28 cases of cystitis.[7]

MICROBIOLOGY

The pathogens responsible for uncomplicated UTIs have been consistent for many years, with *Escherichia coli* the primary pathogen in the vast majority of acute uncomplicated cystitis and most episodes of complicated UTIs and pyelonephritis.[1] *Staphylococcus saprophyticus* accounts for 5% to 15% of UTIs, typically seen in sexually active younger women with acute cystitis.[8] Other gram-negative bacilli, such as Klebsiella and *Proteus mirabilis*, and the gram-positive cocci—enterococcus and group B streptococcus—make up the majority of the remaining cases.[9,10]

Complicated UTIs and catheter-associated UTIs have a wider range of associated pathogens. Polymicrobial infections are encountered more frequently. Resistant organisms, such as extended-spectrum β-lactamase (ESBL), producing enterobacteriaceae, *Pseudomonas aeruginosa,* or *Enterococcus faecium*, are more common in complicated infections. Young men without a history of UTIs typically have a uropathogenic *E coli*. Older men, with a history of obstruction, can have a variety of organisms. If *Staphylococcus aureus* is isolated, a bacteremic source seeding the kidney should be considered.

CLINICAL PRESENTATION

The anatomic location and type of UTI can often be determined by the clinical presentation, but some degree of clinical uncertainty is common in the ED. Acute cystitis is characterized by dysuria and frequent or urgent urination and occurs primarily in healthy, premenopausal, adult women who are not pregnant. These symptoms of urethral irritation can also occur in sexually transmitted infections (STIs), in vaginitis, and with exposure to chemical or allergic irritants. Because UTIs and STIs are both common and may coexist in the same population, it is a frequent differential diagnosis challenge.[11]

Acute pyelonephritis involves the upper urinary tract and is typically associated with systemic symptoms, characterized by fevers, chills, nausea, and flank pain. Patients often also have symptoms of acute cystitis (dysuria, frequency, and urgency). Some patients may describe the pain associated with pyelonephritis in atypical locations, such as the epigastric region or right or left upper abdominal quadrants. Fever is commonly present, and its absence should heighten suspicion for the presence of other clinical conditions. In a retrospective cohort study of women 15 years of age or older admitted to the hospital with the diagnosis of pyelonephritis, those patients lacking fever (temperature less than 37.8–C) were more often found to have other diagnoses, such as cholecystitis, pelvic inflammatory disease, and diverticulitis.[12] The presentation of pyelonephritis can be particularly challenging in the elderly, who may be afebrile or have only a low-grade temperature. They may not be able to verbalize their symptoms (eg, patients with dementia or stroke) and may present with altered mental status, lethargy, or complaints of abdominal pain or generalized weakness.

Uncomplicated UTIs are a disease of reproductive age women. Known risk factors include recent sexual intercourse, the use of spermicides, and a personal history of UTIs. Patients with a history of a UTI are often able to accurately self-diagnose. The 4 symptoms that increase the probability of a UTI are dysuria, frequency, hematuria, and back pain. Having vaginal discharge decreases the probability of a UTI. The combination of dysuria and frequency without vaginal discharge makes the probability of a UTI greater than 90%.[13] These older studies still have not been validated, however.

The distinction between cystitis and pyelonephritis is clinical. Although a diagnosis of pyelonephritis may be obvious in patients with fever and flank pain, many clinical presentations may suggest the possibility of infection involving the kidneys but without certainty. Many women who complain of dysuria and frequency also report subjective fever or vague pain in the back without significant costovertebral angle tenderness. In these circumstances, clinical judgment dictates whether to treat for cystitis (such as with nitrofurantoin) or to give treatment that achieves adequate levels in the kidney tissue and treat pyelonephritis. Older techniques for distinguishing upper tract disease from cystitis, such as a bladder washout with antibiotic solution or detection of antibody-coated bacteria, are never used in practice but have added to knowledge of the subject; it is not uncommon to have subclinical pyelonephritis.[14,15] Patients who are at higher risk for subclinical pyelonephritis include patients with complicating features, such as history of recurrent UTIs; patients with longer duration of symptoms (greater than 7 days); patients who have failed short-course UTI therapy; male patients; and patients with diabetes, pregnancy, or immunosuppression. In clinical practice, the diagnosis of subclinical pyelonephritis is often made in patients who fail a short course of antibiotics for acute cystitis.

LABORATORY DIAGNOSIS

The clinical diagnosis is often not straightforward, and urine testing is usually helpful. This starts with careful collection of urine for urinalysis and possibly a culture. The bladder is normally sterile—urine collected by suprapubic aspiration should not contain leukocytes or bacteria. This is invasive and rarely necessary in clinical practice. The most common method for obtaining urine samples is a clean-catch midstream specimen.[16] In a prospective study of 105 women with UTI symptoms in the ED, there were no statistically significant differences in urinalysis findings or the rate of positive urine cultures when urine was obtained through a midstream clean-catch or in-and-out catheterization.[17] Midstream clean-catch technique can be difficult, however, especially for elderly patients and those with other impairments. Even for those who perform the procedure correctly, surrounding areas can be difficult to clean well. Catherization may be necessary for those who are too ill or immobilized to provide an accurate specimen.

The definitive diagnosis of a UTI is made with a urine culture showing significant bacteriuria. Practically, culture information is not available within the time frame of an ED visit, so diagnosis is based on rapid tests that predict bacteriuria. Several methods are used to evaluate the urine in the clinical laboratory. These include dipstick testing, microscopic examination, and urine flow cytometry. Studies on the utility of these various methods are limited because of varying criteria for defining UTIs.[16] Additionally, leukocytes in the urine occur in both UTIs and noninfectious diseases. Emergency physicians must evaluate the urinalysis in light of these known limitations.

The urine dipstick continues to have a prominent role in the diagnosis of UTI. This test is more convenient and less expensive, and its accuracy in predicting a UTI is comparable to urine microscopy.[18] The dipstick is limited by what it tests. Pyuria is present in the vast majority of patients with acute cystitis and pyelonephritis.[19] There is, however, a wide range of reported sensitivities to detect bacteriuria. Leukocyte esterase has a sensitivity of 62% to 98% and specificity of 55% to 96%. In a systematic review, the urine nitrite was found highly specific.[20] Sensitivity is poor, however, because some pathogens, such as *Staphylococcus saprophyticus* and enterococcus, do not reduce nitrate. A positive test also requires sufficient incubation of the urine in the bladder and nitrate in the patient's diet (vegetables).[21] False-positive results are rare but can occur when urine is discolored (eg severe dehydration or phenazopyridine), making the test difficult to interpret.[22] Furthermore, the interpretation of these tests depends on symptoms.[23] No component of the dipstick can rule out disease in patients with a moderate to high pretest probability.[20]

Patients with classic UTI symptoms occasionally have a negative urinalysis. A common clinical practice in these patients (although not unique to EDs) is to obtain a urine culture, initiate antimicrobial therapy for UTI, and exclude other potential causes for the symptoms (eg, STIs). In a prospective, double-blind, randomized, placebo-controlled trial of 59 women 16 to 50 years of age, presenting with complaints of dysuria and frequency and with a negative urine dipstick test for leukocytes and nitrites, 3 days of antimicrobial therapy significantly reduced dysuria. At the completion of therapy, 76% of patients who received antibiotics reported resolution of dysuria compared with 26% of women in the placebo group ($P = .0005$). At day 7, 90% of the treated women reported resolution of dysuria compared with 59% of women in the placebo group ($P = .02$) (number needed to treat = 4).[24]

Automated instruments perform most of the microscopic analysis in modern hospital laboratories. Some instruments also report the presence of bacteria. The utility of this test may show promise, because these instruments can directly detect bacteria, not just indirect evidence of infection.[25] The absence of bacteria on automated systems should not dissuade clinicians, however, from the diagnosis of UTI if the symptoms are appropriate.

Although urine culture is the reference standard for confirming the diagnosis of UTI, it provides no immediate diagnostic utility in EDs. Urine cultures are recommended in those situations in which they are most likely beneficial, including complicated infections, pyelonephritis, and recent prior antimicrobial treatment.[4] Pretreatment urine cultures are often not performed in patients who present with symptoms of uncomplicated cystitis, where routine cultures have not been shown cost effective or predictive of the therapeutic outcome.[26] These studies were conducted, however, when resistance to standard UTI therapies, such as trimethoprim-sulfamethoxazole and fluoroquinolones, was not as prevalent as today. In the current era of increasing resistance, especially as resistance has been shown to translate into clinical and microbiologic failure, there may be justification for culturing patients with uncomplicated infections.[27,28] It is recognized that a small fraction of uncomplicated cystitis cases may become more complicated as the illness progresses. Hindsight criticism regarding lack of cultures in these cases must be balanced against the recognition that many unnecessary cultures would be required to identify these few. This is an area of reasonable debate and further studies are warranted to optimize use of this resource.

In those cases of cultures sent from the ED, there should be a system for following-up the results or for insuring that results are sent to the appropriate clinicians for follow-up. Because this can be a time-consuming task in a busy department, it is another consideration when deciding whether to send cultures on low-risk patients. This is also a reason the authors do not recommend screening asymptomatic patients for pyuria or bacteruria. Results are often reviewed later by physicians or nurse practitioners with limited access to clinical information. These clinicians may be more likely to recommend unnecessary treatment of a positive culture if the appropriate clinical context is not available, which may lead to undesirable outcomes, such as antimicrobial resistance, adverse drug effects, and cost without benefit.

When culture results demonstrate resistance to the prescribed antimicrobial, patients should be contacted and informed of the result. If symptoms have improved or resolved, it may not be necessary to prescribe a new antimicrobial. Due to high urinary concentrations of many UTI antimicrobials, some infections with demonstrated in vitro resistance may nonetheless be clinically cured. If symptoms have not adequately improved, however, alternate treatment based on susceptibility results should be provided.

Blood cultures have a limited role in the management of most UTIs. Blood culture is virtually never advised for acute cystitis. The role of blood cultures in pyelonephritis is more controversial. Various studies have investigated the utility of blood cultures in patients with pyelonephritis.[29–31] Although patients with pyelonephritis can often be bacteremic, the blood and urine culture results are almost always concordant, and management is not changed. A 7-day course of ciprofloxacin is adequate even in patients with positive blood cultures.[32] Positive blood cultures from skin contaminants are not uncommon and can lead to increased utilization of resources, repeated blood cultures, and prolonged hospitalization. On the basis of the available evidence, it is best to reserve blood cultures for postmenopausal women (for whom cultures are more often discordant), complicated infections, and immunosuppressed patients. Other less common circumstances may also prompt blood cultures. For example, a patient with fever and pyuria but without other symptoms of pyelonephritis could have endocarditis, and blood cultures could be useful.

When blood cultures are obtained, it is again important to have a system to follow-up on the results for patients who have been sent home from an ED. In many cases, pyelonephritis patients are advised to return to the hospital when blood cultures are positive for a typical uropathogen (eg, *E coli*). This is probably unnecessary in most cases. The authors recommend that patients be contacted by telephone to inform them of the results and inquire as to how they are feeling. If symptoms are improved and the organism is susceptible to prescribed antibiotics, then patients can be instructed to complete the course of treatment and return if symptoms worsen or fail to resolve.

IMAGING

There are no specific formal guidelines for the use of imaging studies for patients with UTIs. In most instances, especially in young women with uncomplicated infections, routine radiographic evaluation is not warranted. Underlying structural abnormalities are uncommon, and focal complications rarely occur in this population. Imaging studies may provide insight, however, as to the cause of the symptoms (eg, kidney stone with or without infection) in situations in which there is diagnostic uncertainty (eg, moderate-to-severe illness with low degree of pyuria) or in patients who have failed therapy or present with recurrent infections. Imaging studies are especially valuable in identifying patients who may have lesions requiring surgical correction (eg, renal or extrarenal abscess, emphysematous pyelonephritis, or obstruction).

Early and expedited imaging studies are also recommended in patients who present with UTIs associated with severe sepsis/septic shock. Source control is an essential component of therapy in patients with severe sepsis/septic shock.[33,34] The clinical diagnosis of complications associated with UTI that requires surgical intervention (eg, obstruction, abscess, or emphysematous pyelonephritis) can be difficult, and imaging studies can be critical in revealing these conditions. In practice, the decision to perform an imaging study in the ED setting is most often based on the clinical suspicion of the presence of underlying structural abnormality or other complicating factors (eg, renal or extrarenal abscess, urolithiasis, and emphysematous pyelonephritis). For patients with severe illness, however, the clinical diagnosis of such complications is insufficiently accurate and urgent radiographic evaluation is recommended.

Imaging tests often used in the ED for further evaluation of renal pathologies include plain-film abdominal radiography, ultrasound, and CT scan. Plain-film abdominal radiography (kidneys, ureters, and bladder [KUB]) is of limited use by itself. It may show the presence of renal calculi or gas; however, the sensitivity is lower than that of CT scan and does not demonstrate complications, such as obstruction or hydronephrosis. Plain-film abdominal radiography (KUB) is useful for the rapid evaluation of urinary stent position.

Bedside renal ultrasound is done commonly by many emergency physicians. Emergency medicine residency programs include ultrasound training in their curriculum. Renal ultrasound is a valuable diagnostic tool for the evaluation of acute flank pain, especially in unstable patients who cannot tolerate other diagnostic tests, such as CT scan.[35,36] Ultrasound can reveal complications, such as hydronephrosis, renal or extrarenal abscesses, and distal hydroureter (eg, ureterovesical or uteropelvic junction). **Figs. 1** and **2** show images of bedside ultrasound revealing nephrolithiasis and hydronephrosis. In comparison with CT scan, renal ultrasound is not a good test for the detection of ureteral stones or the evaluation of upper and midureter dilatation.

Helical CT scan, in contrast to renal ultrasound, provides more detailed information and is considered the imaging modality of choice for most renal pathologies in the evaluation of flank pain.[37,38] Noncontrast CT scan accurately localizes the size of urinary calculi, hydroureter at all levels, hydronephrosis, gas, and abscess. The precise localization of gas has important therapeutic and prognostic implications and is crucial for the differentiation of emphysematous pyelonephritis from other conditions, such as emphysematous pyelitis, perinephric emphysema, or abscess. The addition of contrast better enables the delineation of abscess from other structures and can provide insight into renal perfusion and reveal renal infarction, renal artery occlusion, or renal vein thrombosis.

UROLITHIASIS AND UTI

Patients with ureteral stones are commonly treated in EDs because they are in severe pain. The diagnosis of UTI accompanying urolithiasis can be challenging, especially when a patient does not have overt signs of infection. A variable degree of pyuria is frequently encountered in acute presentations of urolithiasis. Whether this finding reflects nonspecific inflammation or true infection is, however, unclear. In a prospective observational study of 360 adult patients presenting with acute urolithiasis, approximately 8% were found to have UTI. Clinical features associated with higher likelihood

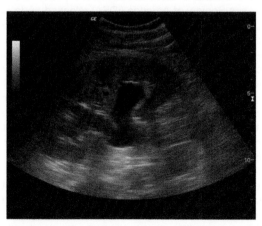

Fig. 1. Hydronephrosis shown on a bedside ultrasound. (*Courtesy of* Michael Stone, MD, Boston, MA.)

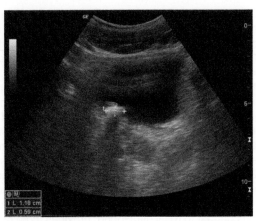

Fig. 2. Bedside ED ultrasound showing a large distal ureterovesical junction stone. (*Courtesy of* Michael Stone, MD, Boston, MA.)

of UTI were female gender, history of dysuria, frequent urination, chills, prior UTI, or fever. Pyuria was only moderately accurate as an indicator of UTI. Pyuria at a cutoff of 5 white blood cells per high-power field was 86% sensitive and 79% specific for UTI. The probability of infection became progressively greater as the level of pyuria increased.[39]

Because of the potential for serious complications (eg, abscess formation, pyonephrosis, and severe sepsis), it is reasonable to initiate antibiotics in patients with urolithiasis who have pyuria regardless of the presence or absence of clinical signs and symptoms of infection. In a study of patients with pyonephrosis associated with nephrolithiasis, a wide spectrum of clinical presentations was found, varying from asymptomatic bacteriuria to urosepsis, including patients without fever or peripheral leukocytosis.[40] Urine cultures can be falsely negative in the presence of an obstructing stone if the infection is proximal to the obstruction.[41]

MANAGEMENT
Uncomplicated Cystitis

The Infectious Diseases Society of America (IDSA) released updated clinical practice guidelines in 2011 for the management of uncomplicated cystitis and pyelonephritis.[3] The recommendations now more emphatically recommend nitrofurantoin, fosfomycin, and trimethoprim-sulfamethoxazole as first-line treatments (**Table 1**). They also emphasize the concept of collateral damage to intestinal and vaginal flora from broad-spectrum antibiotics, highlighting the overuse of fluoroquinolones.

The basic principles that guide recommendations for treatment of cystitis are that antimicrobials should be active against the likely pathogens, should achieve adequate concentrations in the urine, and should have minimal effect on normal flora and that shorter courses are generally associated with lower cost and fewer adverse events. Although cystitis is often a self-resolving infection and cure rates with placebo are as high as 25% to 42%,[3] antimicrobial resistance is associated with greater likelihood of treatment failure. The laboratory cutpoints for resistance attempt to correlate with the urine concentration and, although many antibiotics are concentrated in the urine, the susceptibility tests still correlate with clinical failure rates.

Widespread resistance of coliform bacteria to trimethroprim-sulfamethoxazole has made nitrofurantoin and fosfomycin first-line drugs. Both are effective against *E coli*,

| Table 1 |
| Treatment of uncomplicated cystitis |

Antibiotic	Dosage	Comments
First-line agents		
Nitrofurantoin monohydrate macrocrystals	100 mg PO BID for 5 d	Low rates of resistance. Does not achieve adequate tissue level to treat pyelonephritis. Not recommended in elderly.
Fosfomycin trometamol	3-g Sachet PO × 1 dose	Does not achieve adequate tissue levels to treat pyelonephritis. Possibly inferior to other agents.
Trimethoprim-sulfamethoxazole	(160/800 mg) 1 PO BID for 3 d	Recommended when resistance rates are lower than 20%.
Pivmecillinam	400 mg BID for 3 d	Not available in the United States. Good reported efficacy with minimal ecologic effects.
Second-line agents		
Ciprofloxacin	500 mg PO BID for 3 d	Increasing rates of resistance. Consider using if possible upper tract infection.
Levofloxacin	500 mg PO QD for 3 d	Same as ciprofloxacin.
Cefpodoxime	100 mg PO BID for 5 d	Consider if known resistance to first line agents. β-Lactam agents are generally inferior agents for UTIs.

are well tolerated, and have few ecologic effects.[7] Nitrofurantoin is less active against other pathogens, however, and inactive against Proteus and *Pseudomonas aeruginosa* and, thus, should not be used for empiric therapy for complicated UTIs, in which these organisms are more common. Fosfomycin is appealing for ED use because it can be given as a single dose for simple cystitis and, therefore, does not require that a patient go to the pharmacy. The clinical data on fosfomycin are sparse and single-dose fosfomycin may be inferior to trimethoprim-sulfamethoxazole and ciprofloxacin.[2] *Staphylococcus saprophyticus* remains susceptible to most antibiotics used for UTIs.

Although antimicrobials with high urine concentrations and minimal effects on normal flora (eg, nitrofurantoin) are preferred, emergency physicians may hesitate to use these drugs for patients who have symptoms suggesting possible upper tract disease, such as subjective fever or back pain. Nitrofurantoin and fosfomycin do not achieve adequate blood and tissue levels and are, therefore, not effective for pyelonephritis. These concerns are magnified because emergency physicians generally do not provide longitudinal care and are not able to follow-up patients' symptoms, and this may encourage physicians to use broader-spectrum antibiotics. For these equivocal cases, the authors give ciprofloxacin (500 mg twice daily for 3 days). Patient satisfaction ratings are increasingly used as quality indicators for physicians. Effective initial therapy may be more important to emergency physicians because of the lack of follow-up. A strategy of narrow-spectrum initial treatment with follow-up for alternate treatment of failures is more problematic in the ED setting. Furthermore, repeat visits for the same condition may not be covered by insurance companies.

Despite the 1999 IDSA guidelines for management of UTI, fluoroquinolones were the most commonly prescribed antibiotics for UTI. In 2010, 40.4% of adult patients presenting to US EDs with a primary diagnosis of a UTI received either ciprofloxacin or levofloxacin, representing 1.2 million patients; 13% of patients received trimethoprim-sulfamethoxazole (370,000) and 11% received nitrofurantoin (311,000).[6]

Fluoroquinolones and β-lactam antibiotics are reserved for patients who have failed first-line therapy or have contraindications. Most emergency physicians are not aware that multiple trials have demonstrated that β-lactams are not as effective for UTIs as the other recommended regimens. A recent trial comparing ciprofloxacin and cefpodoxime provides further evidence that even third-generation cephalosporins are not appropriate 3-day regimens.[42]

UTI Versus STI

Another common scenario of diagnostic uncertainty in EDs is making the distinction between UTI and genital STI. Both are common in otherwise healthy individuals of reproductive age, and there is much overlap in the clinical syndromes of dysuria and associated symptoms. In men, the clinical syndromes of prostatitis and epididymitis are known to be caused by either typical uropathogens, such as *E coli*, or by sexually transmitted pathogens, such as *Chlamydia trachomatis* or *Neisseria gonorrhoeae*. In women, dysuria may be a presentation of UTI but can also be a presentation of chlamydia or gonorrhea as well as herpes simplex. Urethritis from any of these pathogens can be associated with pyuria on a clean-catch specimen. Identification of the pathogen by urine culture or by nucleic acid amplification test is generally not available within the time frame of an ED visit.

Clinicians are, therefore, left with the options of providing empiric treatment of UTI, providing empiric treatment of STI, or providing empiric treatment that is active against both possibilities. If clinicians choose to treat for only one possibility, then it is important to follow-up on the results of urine cultures or STI tests so treatment can be provided later if they are positive. Because of the difficulty contacting patients from EDs and having them return for treatment, there is an incentive to provide empiric treatment that covers both possibilities when there is reasonable diagnostic uncertainty. One option is to use levofloxacin, which has activity against common uropathogens as well as chlamydia, with or without an intramuscular dose of ceftriaxone.

Pyelonephritis

Patients with pyelonephritis are frequently quite ill when they present to an ED. Many are in severe pain, febrile, tachycardic, vomiting, and dehydrated, often meeting criteria for sepsis. Nonetheless, a majority can be successfully treated as outpatients if symptomatically improved after a period of observation and treatment in an ED that includes intravenous hydration, antibiotics, antipyretics, and antiemetics. When patients fail to improve in the ED, bedside ultrasound should be considered to rule out ureteral obstruction, perinephric abscess, or other complication. For patients with severe sepsis/septic shock, it is important to provide aggressive fluid resuscitation and use other modalities to optimize tissue oxygen delivery.[33]

Empiric antibiotic recommendations for pyelonephritis are different from those for cystitis for a couple of reasons. Pyelonephritis is more often associated with systemic illness and progression to severe sepsis. It is important to choose therapy that achieves adequate levels not only in the urine but also in renal tissue and blood due to the real possibility of bacteremia. For these reasons, fluoroquinolones are usually the first-line choice, despite concerns about greater likelihood of selecting resistance among intestinal flora (**Table 2**).

Fluoroquinolone resistance has increased greatly in recent years. Although this was largely driven by use of fluoroquinolones for respiratory infections, the greatest impact has been on management of UTIs. In areas where there is more than 10% fluoroquinolone resistance, IDSA guidelines recommend giving a long-acting parenteral antibiotic, such as ceftriaxone. The rationale is that this provides more reliable antimicrobial coverage during the first day while culture and susceptibility results are pending. In a study of trimethoprim-sulfamethoxazole versus ciprofloxacin for pyelonephritis patients in an ED, cure rates were significantly higher in patients with organisms resistant to the oral antibiotic when they were given an initial dose of ceftriaxone.[43]

In addition to increasing resistance to trimethoprim-sulfamethoxazole and fluoroquinolones, uropathogens producing ESBL are also becoming more common.[44–47] Although they are more common in many other countries, they are now emerging in some areas of the United States.[48] In areas in which ESBLs are found, clinicians may consider initial empiric treatment with a carbapenem for UTI associated with severe sepsis or septic shock. Patients with uncomplicated pyelonephritis can be treated with a 7-day course of oral ciprofloxacin, even if they are found bacteremic.[3,32,43] Alternate treatments should be considered if there is a history of infection with resistant organisms.

Complicated Urinary Tract Infections

It is difficult to make overall recommendations on complicated UTIs because of the broad range of complicating factors and associated pathogens. Because the bacteriology of complicated infections is more diverse and antimicrobial resistance more common, it is especially important to obtain culture specimens in these cases. Not surprisingly, there are no published consensus guidelines for these circumstances, and the vast amount of literature on UTIs deals with uncomplicated UTIs. Some

Table 2
Treatment of uncomplicated pyelonephritis[a]

Antibiotic	Dosage	Comments
First-line agents		
Ciprofloxacin	500 mg PO BID for 7 d	Fluoroquinolones are the drug of choice for pyelonephritis despite ecologic adverse effects. There is increasing resistance, however, of E coli to these agents
Levofloxacin	750 mg PO QD for 5 d	Same as for ciprofloxacin.
Second-line agents		
Cefpodoxime	200 mg PO BID for 10–14 d	Minimal evidence on using cefpodoxime or other β-lactam agents for pyelonephritis.
Trimethoprim-sulfamethoxazole	(160/800 mg) 1 PO BID for 14 d	Give ceftriaxone or aminoglycocide.

[a] An initial dose of 1 g of ceftriaxone or once-a-day dose of gentamicin (5–7 mg per kg) is recommended if using second-line agents or if there is greater than 10% resistance of E coli to fluoroquinolone.

patients who are classically grouped as having complicated infections, such as those with controlled diabetes or postmenopausal women, can usually be treated the same as those with uncomplicated infections.

One complicated UTI scenario commonly encountered in the ED is the presence of an indwelling urinary catheter, in which diagnosis of UTI can be challenging. Depending on the duration of catheterization, most catheterized patients have bacteriuria often accompanied with pyuria. Hence, on the basis of urinalysis, the distinction between those who are merely colonized and those who have a "true" infection is not straightforward.[49] Because culture results are not available during ED evaluation, emergency physicians rely on the presence of clinical signs and symptoms of infection to diagnose catheter-associated UTI. This approach has its pitfalls, however. Most patients with indwelling urinary catheters who present to the ED are elderly and residing in nursing homes. These patients frequently have multiple medical problems, are on numerous medications, and are usually not able to verbalize their symptoms. In addition, they may lack clinical signs of infection and often present with an altered level of consciousness. Another pitfall is attributing the source of infection to the urine and overlooking other causes (eg, pneumonia or ischemic bowel). Because catheter-associated UTI is a common cause of nosocomial morbidity and mortality, empiric antimicrobial therapy, in addition to replacement or removal of the catheter, is often appropriate in such patients.

DISPOSITION

Probably the single most important decision made in the ED is whether a patient is admitted to the hospital or sent home. This decision has a great impact on cost—outpatient treatment of UTI typically costs 10s of dollars, but inpatient treatment costs 1000s. Cost must be balanced against the need for specialized inpatient services and the risk of rapid deterioration at home that may not be adequately addressed by return precautions. Although there are validated decision rules to inform admission decisions for some other infections, such as pneumonia, there is no validated decision rule to determine who gets admitted for UTI. **Box 2** lists some common indications for admission.

Many patients with pyelonephritis initially appear toxic with high fevers, vomiting, and tachycardia, but their symptoms can improve quickly in an ED with antipyretics, intravenous fluids, antiemetics, and antibiotics. Most can then be discharged home with oral antibiotics. With increasing fluoroquinolone resistance, it is especially important to follow-up on culture and susceptibility results after patients are discharged home.

Box 2
Possible indications for admission for patients with pyelonephritis
Intractable nausea or vomiting
Hemodynamic instability
Presence of obstruction or complications (emphysematous pyelonephritis)
Failure of outpatient therapy
Poor social support (inability to purchase medications or obtain follow-up)
Suspicion of resistant organism with no oral treatment option

Because of the potential for both maternal and fetal complications, pregnant women with pyelonephritis are most often admitted to the hospital (at least for a brief period of observation) and treated with intravenous antibiotics. Oral outpatient therapy has been shown safe and effective for the treatment of selected pregnant patients with pyelonephritis.[50,51] These studies included initial observation and treatment with parenteral antibiotics; however, no outpatient trials have been done in pregnant patients in whom oral therapy was used alone.

SUMMARY

Emergency physicians encounter UTIs in a wide spectrum of disease severity and patient populations. Unusual presentations are common, and some patients may lack the classic symptoms of UTI. The diagnosis is especially challenging in the elderly, patients with indwelling catheters, and in patients with acute urolithiasis. Most patients do not require an extensive diagnostic evaluation and can be safely managed as outpatients with oral antibiotics.

REFERENCES

1. Stamm WE, Hooton TM. Management of urinary-tract infections in adults. N Engl J Med 1993;329(18):1328–34.
2. Warren JW, Abrutyn E, Hebel JR, et al. Guidelines for antimicrobial treatment of uncomplicated acute bacterial cystitis and acute pyelonephritis in women. Clin Infect Dis 1999;29(4):745–58.
3. Gupta K, Hooton TM, Naber KG, et al. International clinical practice guidelines for the treatment of acute uncomplicated cystitis and pyelonephritis in women: a 2010 update by the Infectious Diseases Society of America and the European Society for Microbiology and Infectious Diseases. Clin Infect Dis 2011;52(5): E103–20.
4. Neal DE. Complicated urinary tract infections. Urol Clin North Am 2008;35(1): 13–22.
5. HCUPnet. Healthcare cost and utilization project (HCUP). Rockville (MD): Agency for Healthcare Research and Quality; 2010. Available at: http://hcupnet.hhrq.gov/. Accessed July 4, 2013.
6. National Center for Health Statistics. National hospital ambulatory medical care survey (NHAMCS), 2010. Hyattsville (MD). Public-use data file and documentation. Available at: ftp://ftp.cdc.gov/pub/Health_Statistics/NCHS/Datasets/NHAMCS/. Accessed August 2, 2013.
7. Hooton TM. Uncomplicated urinary tract infection. N Engl J Med 2012;366(11): 1028–37.
8. Jordan PA, Iravani A, Richard GA, et al. Urinary-tract infection caused by Staphylococcus-saprophyticus. J Infect Dis 1980;142(4):510–5.
9. Talan DA, Krishnadasan A, Abrahamian FM, et al. Prevalence and risk factor analysis of trimethoprim-sulfamethoxazole- and fluoroquinolone-resistant Escherichia coli infection among emergency department patients with pyelonephritis. Clin Infect Dis 2008;47(9):1150–8.
10. Gupta K, Sahm DF, Mayfield D, et al. Antimicrobial resistance among uropathogens that cause community-acquired urinary tract infections in women: a nationwide analysis. Clin Infect Dis 2001;33(1):89–94.
11. Shapiro T, Dalton M, Hammock J, et al. The prevalence of urinary tract infections and sexually transmitted disease in women with symptoms of a simple urinary

tract infection stratified by low colony count criteria. Acad Emerg Med 2005; 12(1):38–44.

12. Pinson AG, Philbrick JT, Lindbeck GH, et al. Fever in the clinical diagnosis of acute pyelonephritis. Am J Emerg Med 1997;15(2):148–51.

13. Bent S, Nallamothu BK, Simel DL, et al. Does this woman have an acute uncomplicated urinary tract infection? JAMA 2002;287(20):2701–10.

14. Fairley KF, Carson NE, Gutch RC, et al. Site of infection in acute urinary tract infection in general practice. Lancet 1971;2(7725):615–8.

15. Jones SR, Smith JW, Sanford JP. Localization of urinary-tract infections by detection of antibody-coated bacteria in urine sediment. N Engl J Med 1974; 290(11):591–3.

16. Wilson ML, Gaido L. Laboratory diagnosis of urinary tract infections in adult patients. Clin Infect Dis 2004;38(8):1150–8.

17. Walter FG, Knopp RK. Urine sampling in ambulatory women - midstream clean-catch versus catherization. Ann Emerg Med 1989;18(2):166–72.

18. Lammers RL, Gibson S, Kovacs D, et al. Comparison of test characteristics of urine dipstick and urinalysis at various test cutoff points. Ann Emerg Med 2001;38(5):505–12.

19. Stamm WE. Measurement of pyuria and its relation to bacteriuria. Am J Med 1983;75(1B):53–8.

20. Meister L, Morley EJ, Scheer D, et al. History and physical examination plus laboratory testing for the diagnosis of adult female urinary tract infection. Acad Emerg Med 2013;20(7):631–45.

21. Aspevall O, Hallander H, Gant V, et al. European guidelines for urinalysis: a collaborative document produced by European clinical microbiologists and clinical chemists under ECLM in collaboration with ESCMID. Clin Microbiol Infect 2001;7(4):173–8.

22. Roy JB, Wilkerson RG. Fallability of Griess (Nitrite) test. Urology 1984;23(3): 270–1.

23. Lachs MS, Nachamkin I, Edelstein PH, et al. Spectrum bias in the evaluation of diagnostic tests - lessons learned from the rapid dipstick test for urinary-tract infection. Ann Intern Med 1992;117(2):135–40.

24. Richards D, Toop L, Chambers S, et al. Response to antibiotics of women with symptoms of urinary tract infection but negative dipstick urine test results: double blind randomised controlled trial. BMJ 2005;331(7509):143B–6B.

25. Jiang T, Chen PS, Ouyang JA, et al. Urine particles analysis: performance evaluation of Sysmex UF-1000i and comparison among urine flow cytometer, dipstick, and visual microscopic examination. Scand J Clin Lab Invest 2011; 71(1):30–7.

26. Carlson KJ, Mulley AG. Management of acute dysuria - a decision-analysis model of alternative strategies. Ann Intern Med 1985;102(2):244–9.

27. Abrahamian FM, Krishnadasan A, Mower WR, et al. The association of antimicrobial resistance with cure and quality of life among women with acute uncomplicated cystitis. Infection 2011;39(6):507–14.

28. Raz R, Chazan B, Kennes Y, et al. Empiric use of trimethoprim-sulfamethoxazole (TMP-SMX) in the treatment of women with uncomplicated urinary tract infections, in a geographical area with a high prevalence of TMP-SMX-resistant uropathogens. Clin Infect Dis 2002;34(9):1165–9.

29. Velasco M, Martinez JA, Moreno-Martinez A, et al. Blood cultures for women with uncomplicated acute pyelonephritis: are they necessary? Clin Infect Dis 2003; 37(8):1127.

30. Chen Y, Nitzan O, Saliba W, et al. Are blood cultures necessary in the management of women with complicated pyelonephritis? J Infect 2006;53(4):235–40.
31. Hsu CY, Fang HC, Chou KJ, et al. The clinical impact of bacteremia in complicated acute pyelonephritis. Am J Med Sci 2006;332(4):175–80.
32. Sandberg T, Skoog G, Hermansson AB, et al. Ciprofloxacin for 7 days versus 14 days in women with acute pyelonephritis: a randomised, open-label and double-blind, placebo-controlled, non-inferiority trial. Lancet 2012;380(9840):484–90.
33. Nguyen HB, Rivers EP, Abrahamian FM, et al. Severe sepsis and septic shock: review of the literature and emergency department management guidelines. Ann Emerg Med 2006;48(1):28–54.
34. Talan DA, Moran GJ, Abrahamian FM. Severe sepsis and septic shock in the emergency department. Infect Dis Clin North Am 2008;22(1):1–31.
35. Gaspari RJ, Horst K. Emergency ultrasound and urinalysis in the evaluation of flank pain. Acad Emerg Med 2005;12(12):1180–4.
36. Kartal M, Eray O, Erdogru T, et al. Prospective validation of a current algorithm including bedside US performed by emergency physicians for patients with acute flank pain suspected for renal colic. Emerg Med J 2006;23(5):341–4.
37. Jindal G, Ramchandani P. Acute flank pain secondary to urolithiasis: radiologic evaluation and alternate diagnoses. Radiol Clin North Am 2007;45(3):395–410.
38. Sheafor DH, Hertzberg BS, Freed KS, et al. Nonenhanced helical CT and US in the emergency evaluation of patients with renal colic: prospective comparison. Radiology 2000;217(3):792–7.
39. Abrahamian FM, Krishnadasan A, Mower WR, et al. Association of pyuria and clinical characteristics with the presence of urinary tract infection among patients with acute nephrolithiasis. Ann Emerg Med 2013;62(5):526–33.
40. Stlezin M, Hofmann R, Stoller ML. Pyonephrosis - diagnosis and treatment. Br J Urol 1992;70(4):360–3.
41. Mariappan P, Loong CW. Midstream urine culture and sensitivity test is a poor predictor of infected urine proximal to the obstructing ureteral stone or infected stones: a prospective clinical study. J Urol 2004;171(6):2142–5.
42. Hooton TM, Roberts PL, Stapleton AE. Cefpodoxime vs ciprofloxacin for short-course treatment of acute uncomplicated cystitis a randomized trial. JAMA 2012;307(6):583–9.
43. Talan DA, Stamm WE, Hooton TM, et al. Comparison of ciprofloxacin (7 days) and trimethoprim-sulfamethoxazole (14 days) for acute uncomplicated pyelonephritis in women - a randomized trial. JAMA 2000;283(12):1583–90.
44. Schito GC, Naber KG, Botto H, et al. The ARESC study: an international survey on the antimicrobial resistance of pathogens involved in uncomplicated urinary tract infections. Int J Antimicrob Agents 2009;34(5):407–13.
45. Hoban DJ, Lascols C, Nicolle LE, et al. Antimicrobial susceptibility of Enterobacteriaceae, including molecular characterization of extended-spectrum beta-lactamase-producing species, in urinary tract isolates from hospitalized patients in North America and Europe: results from the SMART study 2009-2010. Diagn Microbiol Infect Dis 2012;74(1):62–7.
46. Meier S, Weber R, Zbinden R, et al. Extended-spectrum beta-lactamase-producing Gram-negative pathogens in community-acquired urinary tract infections: an increasing challenge for antimicrobial therapy. Infection 2011;39(4):333–40.
47. Foxman B. Extended-spectrum beta-lactamase-producing escherichia coli in the united states: time to rethink empirical treatment for suspected E-coli infections? Clin Infect Dis 2013;56(5):649–51.

48. Doi Y, Park YS, Rivera JI, et al. Community-associated extended-spectrum beta-lactamase-producing Escherichia coli infection in the United States. Clin Infect Dis 2013;56(5):641–8.
49. Maki DG, Tambyah PA. Engineering out the risk for infection with urinary catheters. Emerg Infect Dis 2001;7(2):342–7.
50. Millar LK, Wing DA, Paul RH, et al. Outpatient treatment of pyelonephritis in pregnancy - a randomized controlled trial. Obstet Gynecol 1995;86(4):560–4.
51. Wing DA, Hendershott CM, Debuque L, et al. Outpatient treatment of acute pyelonephritis in pregnancy after 24 weeks. Obstet Gynecol 1999;94(5):683–8.

Management of Urinary Tract Infections from Multidrug-Resistant Organisms

Kalpana Gupta, MD, MPH[a,b,]*, Nahid Bhadelia, MD, MA[c]

KEYWORDS

- Multidrug-resistant organisms • Cystitis • Extended-spectrum β-lactamases
- Carbapenem-resistant Enterobacteriaceae • Vancomycin-resistant *Enterococcus*

KEY POINTS

- Antimicrobial resistance to a broad spectrum of agents is encountered with increasing frequency among uropathogens, even in the community setting.
- An understanding of resistance mechanisms and determinants can help optimize empiric therapy.
- Treatment of urinary tract infections from multidrug-resistant organisms is complicated by limited oral options and may require a return to older antibiotics, combination therapy, or intravenous agents.

INTRODUCTION

Infections with antibiotic-resistant pathogens are associated with high morbidity and mortality, and increased cost of hospitalization.[1] Vancomycin-resistant *Enterococcus* blood stream infections decrease survival from 59% to 24% and increase hospital stay from 16.7 to 34.8 days.[2,3] Similar data are available for infections with gram-negatives and methicillin-resistant *Staphylococcus aureus*.[2,4]

Management of patients with infections in the ambulatory setting is particularly challenging because of the increase in resistance among gram-negative bacteria and lack of oral treatment options. Multidrug-resistant pathogens, such as extended-spectrum β-lactamase (ESBL)–producing *Escherichia coli* are now occurring in patients with no

Funding: None.
Conflict of Interest: Dr K. Gupta has served as a consultant to Paratek Pharmaceuticals and holds equity in Aegis Women's Health Technologies; Dr N. Bhadelia: None.
[a] Infectious Diseases, VA Boston HCS, 1400 VFW Parkway, West Roxbury, MA 02312, USA;
[b] Infectious Diseases, Boston University School of Medicine, Dowling 3 North Room 3104, Boston, MA 02115, USA; [c] Section of Infectious Diseases, Boston Medical Center, Boston University School of Medicine, Dowling 3 North Room 3104, Boston, MA 02115, USA
* Corresponding author. Infectious Diseases, 1400 VFW Parkway, VA Boston HCS, MED 111, West Roxbury, MA 02132, USA.
E-mail address: kalpana.gupta@va.gov

discernable health care exposure or risk factors.[5] Microbial resistance has also heralded the need for use of older antibiotics that are known to have significant adverse effects.[6] A recent study of Veterans Administration medical centers showed an increase over a 5-year period in use of broad-spectrum antibiotics, such as polymyxin and tigecycline, for both empiric and targeted therapy.[6]

Recognition and appropriate management of patients with multidrug-resistant urinary tract infections (UTIs) is critical for optimizing outcomes and minimizing cost and inconvenience.

EPIDEMIOLOGY

Antimicrobial resistance among uropathogens has been widely documented. Resistance to commonly used antimicrobials, even in community-associated uncomplicated cystitis, has been described for more than a decade.[7] However, the prevalence of multidrug-resistant organisms in the outpatient setting is increasing, and the problem of uncomplicated UTIs requiring intravenous therapy because of the lack of oral options is a new challenge for clinicians, complicating a once simple-to-treat infection.

The relative frequency of resistant organisms varies by patient population and geography. In cohorts from 5 states, 3.9% of the E coli UTI isolates were positive for ESBL and of those, 36% were from outpatient clinics.[5] Escherichia coli strains that produce CTX-M ESBLs, primarily found in community sources, are becoming widely prevalent worldwide, most notably in Europe and Canada.[8–10] The emergence of these resistance patterns is concerning, particularly in community-onset UTIs, because they are mostly resistant to oral antibiotics.[11–17] One study from Spain reported a 3-fold increase in community-onset UTIs caused by ESBL-producing E coli over a 3-year period, most of which were also resistant to trimethoprim-sulfamethoxazole and fluoroquinolones.[11] Another study from the United Kingdom revealed a similar trend, with 24% of 291 CTX-M–producing E coli isolates (mostly urinary in origin) came from the community. Most of isolates were also resistant to fluoroquinolones, trimethoprim-sulfamethoxazole, and tetracycline.[17] Resistance to commonly prescribed oral antibiotics leads to inadequate empiric therapy and potential development of more severe infections, including bacteremia. A series of nonhospitalized patients with UTIs secondary to ESBL-producing E coli strains showed that 5 of 37 patients became bacteremic, requiring hospitalization because of treatment with inadequate initial empiric therapy.[15] In one study, 4.1% of community-onset bacteremias were caused by ESBL-producing E coli, and these were associated with a mortality rate of 21.1%.[18]

Carbapenem-resistant Enterobacteriaceae (CRE) were uncommon in the United States before 2000. However, the percentage of publically reported CRE increased from 1.2% in 2001 to 4.2% in 2011. Within the United States, the number of facilities reporting CRE was 3 times greater in the Northeast than in the South, Midwest, and West (9.6% vs 3.3%, 3.2%, and 3.6%, respectively).[19] Large metropolitan areas display a disproportionate amount of CRE; almost 21% of Klebsiella pneumoniae isolates from New York City hospitals were reported to be carbapenem-resistant.[20] Hospitals that are of larger size or have an affiliation with a medical school were also associated with higher prevalence of CRE.[19] The scope of CREs has also increased; the New Delhi metallo-β-lactamase 1 (NDM-1) CREs largely ascribed to the Indian subcontinent are now seen in all areas except South and Central America.[21]

Among gram-positives, Enterococcus faecium accounts for most vancomycin-resistant enterococci (VRE) isolates (88%).[22,23] Rates of up to 30% of VRE have been reported in intensive care units in the United States, and the increase in VRE is correlated with the relative prevalence of *E faecium*.[23] An increase in inpatient prevalence is worrisome, because it translates into higher rates of VRE colonization in discharged patients. Forty percent of patients with VRE continue to carry the organism during the first year after hospitalization, and almost a quarter are still colonized by the end of 4 years.[24]

DETERMINANTS OF RESISTANCE

Microbial resistance can be a result of sporadic chromosomal mutations that offer selective advantage and allow organisms to either change the drug target site, increase drug efflux, or limit drug entry. Resistance can also be carried on foreign DNA through transposons and plasmids, which can be transferred between organisms of the same species or across species. Plasmids may also concurrently carry genes for resistance to multiple antibiotics. Hence, multiclass resistance is not uncommon, even among patients only exposed to one class of antimicrobials.

The main pathogens implicated in community-onset UTIs are *E coli*, followed by *Klebsiella* spp and *Proteus* spp. *Escherichia coli* causes 80% of UTIs worldwide.

Gram-negative organisms achieve resistance to β-lactam antibiotics through expression of β-lactamase enzymes, which split the amide bond of the β-lactam ring. The β-lactamases can be carried on chromosomes or as transferable genes.[25] AmpC β-lactamases are carried chromosomally and infer inducible resistance during antibiotic exposure to penicillins, narrow-spectrum cephalosporins and cephamycins, in addition to being resistant to β-lactams. This enzyme is expressed in *Enterobacter*, *Citrobacter freundii*, *Serratia*, *Morganella morganii*, *Providencia*, and *Pseudomonas aeruginosa*.[25]

Enterobacteriaceae also exhibit a class of plasmid-based enzymes that have the ability to inactivate all cephalosporins. These enzymes were initially reported in *K pneumoniae* and *E coli*, but are now noted in other gram-negative species. These extended-spectrum β-lactamases, which were initially selected for in the inpatient setting because of frequent use of cephalosporins, are now increasingly being encountered in the community setting.

Enterobacteriaceae that produce CTX-M β-lactamases, which are the most commonly encountered ESBL isolates in the outpatient setting, also carry concurrent resistance genes to fluoroquinolones, aminoglycosides, and sulfonamides, severely reducing oral treatment options. This cross-resistance is especially prominent in urinary isolates.[26]

Carbapenemases infer the ability to neutralize carbapenems in addition to penicillins and cephalosporins. *Klebsiella pneumonia* carbapenemase (KPC) and NDM-1 are the most clinically relevant enzymes in this class. Carbapenemases were first encountered in *K pneumonia* but are now present throughout this family of Enterobacteriaceae (CRE) and are also seen in other gram-negative bacteria, such as *P aeruginosa*.[21]

Among gram-positive organisms, *Enterococcus* spp and *Staphylococcus saprophyticus* can also cause UTIs. Little resistance is encountered among *S saprophyticus*, because most remain susceptible to multiple antimicrobials.[27] However, resistance among enterococci is a well-known phenomenon with significant clinical consequences. *Enterococcus* is the third most common nosocomial infection, and UTIs are the most frequent infections caused by this pathogen. It may be encountered in patients with recent hospitalization or other exposure to health care–related facilities. Because of their low virulence, enterococci usually affect debilitated hosts or can be found in those with indwelling urinary catheters. They require higher concentrations of penicillin than streptococci, under which they were initially classified. Enterococci are intrinsically resistant to cephalosporins, antistaphylococcal penicillins, trimethoprim, and low concentrations of clindamycin and aminoglycosides. *Enterococcus* spp are now noted to have developed resistance to high concentrations of aminoglycosides, β-lactams, and, most notably, glycopeptides such as vancomycin.[23]

Penicillinase-based resistance is well documented in enterococcal species, as is penicillin resistance derived from mutations in penicillin-binding surface proteins. *Enterococcus faecium* also expresses β-lactamase–based resistance. Resistance to vancomycin can be coded by 6 genes, Van A, B, D, E, G, and L, that downregulate the production of D-alanine–D-alanine, which vancomycin binds to for cell entry. These genes are particularly worrisome, because they can be transferred between enterococci and other species, such as *S aureus* via plasmid or conjugation, increasing the prevalence of vancomycin-resistant staphylococcal strains in coinfected patients.[28]

CLINICAL IMPLICATIONS

At initial presentation, patients should be evaluated for known risk factors for multidrug-resistant bacterial infections in general. These factors include age older than 60 years, prior UTI history or chronic medical conditions, recent hospitalizations or antibiotic treatment, and recent travel.[21] Aside from selection pressure from antimicrobial use, particularly with β-lactam antibiotics and fluoroquinolones, transmission risk factors for ESBL UTIs are not well understood.[5,29,30]

Identifying patients who are colonized versus those who have a clinical infection is a challenge in treating any UTI. In the case of infections with multidrug-resistant organisms, this dilemma is particularly precarious, because treatment presents additional risks of increasing resistance at the population level and narrowing future treatment options for the affected patient. Having said this, the definition of *cystitis*, namely bacteriuria and clinical symptoms, remains consistent regardless of the resistance pattern of the organism. Thus, patients who have asymptomatic bacteriuria should not be treated simply because they carry a multidrug-resistant organism. See the article by Trautner and Grigoryan elsewhere in this issue for an in-depth review of the approach to a positive urine culture in patients without urinary symptoms.

The treatment of true infections with multidrug-resistant organisms requires additional clinical reflection regarding which of the few remaining antibiotics with activity should be chosen, whether single or combination therapy is warranted, and when to hospitalize or switch to intravenous antimicrobial treatment for sicker patients (these patients require closer observation and follow-up). Clinicians and patients need to accept that the initial empiric treatment choice may be incorrect and a switch in therapy may be needed, depending on full susceptibility results and the clinical response.

For uncomplicated cystitis secondary to ESBL organisms, treatment options involve a return to UTI-specific antibiotics, such fosfomycin and nitrofurantoin. Auer and colleagues[31] examined 100 ESBL-producing *E coli* from urinary samples and found high rates of coresistance with other antimicrobials, such as aminoglycosides, fluoroquinolones, and trimethoprim/sulfamethoxazole. The isolates retained high rates of susceptibility to fosfomycin, nitrofurantoin, and ertapenem. A guide to potential therapeutic agents for ESBL-carrying organisms, CRE, and VRE are presented in **Table 1**.

Fosfomycin is a cell wall inhibitor and a bactericidal antibiotic with broad-spectrum activity that has excellent activity in the urinary tract. A recent meta-analysis illustrated the noninferiority of fosfomycin to comparators in clinical outcomes, such as eradication of infection, relapse, and reinfection.[32] Resistance to fosfomycin is uncommon;

Table 1	
Suggested treatment regimens for UTIs secondary to multidrug-resistant organisms	
Organism	**Recommended Treatment Regimens[a]**
ESBL	Uncomplicated: Fosfomycin, 3 g po sachet in 3–4 oz of water × 1 Nitrofurantoin, 100 mg po bid Cefdinir, 300 mg po bid, AND amoxicillin/clavulanic acid, 875 mg po bid (in vitro data only) When susceptibilities are known or local antibiogram is supportive: Trimethoprim/sulfamethoxazole 1 DS tablet po bid Fluoroquinolones (500 mg po bid for ciprofloxacin or 500 mg po daily levofloxacin) Complicated: Cefepime, 2 g IV q12h Ertapenem, 1 g IV per d (other carbapenems also acceptable) Aminoglycosides IV (amikacin, 15–20 mg/kg per d; gentamicin, 4–7 mg/kg per d)
CRE	Aminoglycosides (amikacin, 15–20 mg/kg IV per d; gentamycin, 4–7 mg/kg IV per d) Tigecycline, 100 mg IV as first dose and then 50 mg daily thereafter Polymyxin B, 2 mg/kg IV daily Severe: Consider combination therapy, such as aminoglycoside OR polymyxin B OR tigecycline B, AND carbapenem
VRE	Uncomplicated: Fosfomycin, 3 g po sachet in 3–4 oz of water × 1 Nitrofurantoin, 100 mg po bid Fluoroquinolones (500 mg po bid for ciprofloxacin or 500 mg po daily for levofloxacin) Doxycycline, 100 mg po bid Complicated: Ampicillin, 1–2 g IV q4h and gentamicin, 1 mg/kg IV q8h or streptomycin for synergy (*Enterococcus faecalis*) Linezolid, 600 mg po/IV bid Daptomycin, 4–6 mg/kg IV q24h Tigecycline, 100 mg IV as first dose, and then 50 mg daily thereafter Quinupristin/dalfopristin, 7.5 mg/kg IV q8h (*Enterococcus faecium* only)

Abbreviations: DS, double-strength; IV, intravenous; per d, per day.

[a] Doses based on normal renal function; doses may need adjustment for reduced Glomerular Filtration Rate (GFR). Some studies have used higher doses than those listed herein. Some of the recommendations in this table are not uses approved by the U.S. Food and Drug Administration, but are based on references listed in the text.

Data from Refs.[21,23,35,41,44]

this antibiotic is well tolerated and has few drug interactions, making it a useful choice in this population. However, resistance has increased with its increasing use in some populations.[33]

Nitrofurantoin can achieve good urine and bladder concentrations, but does not achieve adequate serum or tissue levels to serve as treatment for pyelonephritis, prostatitis, or other severe disease. It is also contraindicated in pregnancy and patients with renal failure. Pivmecillinam can also serve as an oral option for uncomplicated infections but should be avoided in ascending infections and is not available in the United States. Other oral antibiotics, such as fluoroquinolones and trimethoprim/sulfamethoxazole, can be used in patients with anticipated susceptibility and when local resistance patterns are known. Where population resistance levels exceed 20%, empiric trimethoprim/sulfamethoxazole should be avoided.[34]

Combination strategy can also be considered with oral agents such as cefdinir, a third-generation cephalosporin and amoxicillin/clavulanic acid. This combination was shown to be active against ESBL producers in vitro, but clinical data on efficacy are not available.[35] In clinical situations requiring intravenous therapy, cefepime and carbapenems should be considered.[36] Ertapenem, with its once-a-day dosing, would be most convenient for outpatient treatment.[37]

Treatment choices for CREs are even more constricted. Furthermore, some of the active agents against CREs such as tigecycline and polymyxin do not have good clearance in the urine. Renal clearance of tigecyline in a patient with normal renal function is noted to be 10% to 20%, and its use in urosepsis is limited to case reports.[38–41] Polymyxin B urinary excretion is even lower, because only 4% of is excreted unchanged in the urine. Neither drug is approved by the U.S. Food and Drug Administration for the treatment of UTIs. A recent retrospective review showed that aminoglycosides are more effective in clearing bacteriuria than polymyxin B or tigecycline. The microbiological clearance rate was 88% in the aminoglycoside group, compared with 64% and 43% in the polymyxin B and tigecycline cohorts, respectively.[41] However, tigecycline and polymyxin B do not seem to require renal adjustment, and hence may have a role in patients with renal dysfunction.[39,42] In severe disease, the use of each of these antimicrobials with a second agent, including carbapenems, seems to result in fewer treatment failures, but the efficacy of different combinations requires further clinical research.[43,44] Case reports also show some success with combination therapy, including colistin and tigecycline.[43]

Like gram-negatives, discerning between colonization and infection can be difficult in the case of VRE. Given its low pathogenicity, this organism can often be a colonizer and result in asymptomatic bacteriuria. Treatment should be considered in those that have clinical signs and symptoms consistent with an infection, or in patients with underlying malignancy or organ transplantation. As many of the vancomycin-resistant Enterococcus faecalis isolates remain sensitive to ampicillin, amoxicillin can be a good oral choice for uncomplicated cystitis. Nitrofurantoin and fosfomycin are 2 other oral options that have been shown to be active against vancomycin-resistant E faecalis in the urine.[23,45,46] Fluoroquinolones also have high urine clearance and are well tolerated. Prior studies have shown E faecalis clearance rates of 71%, 73%, and 79% for gatifloxacin at 200 or 400 mg, and ciprofloxacin at 500 mg twice a day.[23,47] Doxycycline have low levels of urine clearance despite showing activity against VRE, and hence may be of limited utility for treating UTIs.[48]

In patients requiring intravenous antibiotics, ampicillin in conjunction with gentamycin can be considered for ampicillin-susceptible enterococci.[22] Other options for more severe disease are linezolid, daptomycin, tigecycline, and, for E faecium only, quinipristin/dalfopristin.[23] Linezolid is a bacteriostatic antibiotic that inhibits protein synthesis with good renal excretion and has been shown to have an 85% eradication rate for E faecalis. However, linezolid resistance is emerging, and in some institutions has been documented to be as high as 20%.[49,50]

NEW THERAPIES IN THE PIPELINE

Several new approaches are being evaluated to address the dearth of active agents against carbapenemases. In particular, several novel β-lactamase inhibitors with activity against carbapenemases show promise when used in combination with β-lactam agents.[51] Although these agents may have limited activity alone, they potentiate the effect of other β-lactams, extended-spectrum cephalosporins, and aztreonam.

Table 2
Novel β-lactamase inhibitors in combination therapy

β-Lactamase Inhibitor	Agents Used in Combination	Active Against	Reference
Avibactam	Piperacillin, ceftoxime, ceftazidime, cefepime, aztreonam	Klebsiella pneumoniae carbapenemases: K pneumoniae, Pseudomonas aeruginosa	Endimiani et al,[52] 2009; Zhanel et al,[57] 2013
ME1071	Imipenem, biapenem, doripenem, ceftazidime	Class B carbapenemases: P aeruginosa	Ishii et al,[56] 2010
MK-7655	Imipenem	K pneumoniae carbapenemases: K pneumoniae and P aeruginosa	Hirsch et al,[54] 2012
RPX7009	Biapenem	Class A, B, and C carbapenemases: Enterobacteriaceae	Livermore & Mushtaq,[51] 2013

Some promising regimens are presented in **Table 2**.[51–57] Ceftolozane (CXA-101, Cubist Pharmaceuticals, Lexington, MA), serving as a partner antibiotic to the more traditional β-lactam agent, tazobactam, is being evaluated for the indication of pyelo-nephritis and is currently in phase 3 trials. This combination is noted to provide good coverage for P aeruginosa and other ESBL-carrying organisms. It has limited action against Acinetobacter baumannii.[58,59] Plazomicin (AHCN-490), a neoglycoside with phase 2 data, provides coverage for a broad spectrum of fluoroquinolone- and some aminoglycoside-resistant organisms, ESBL-producing pathogens, and CRE. It has limited activity against Proteus spp, and few data with P aeruginosa and A bau-mannii.[58,60] Overall, some organisms remain wholly uncovered. Boucher and col-leagues[58] remark that no drugs have reliable action against A baumannii, and few can withstand metallo-carbapenemases. This article raises appropriate concern regarding the need for further drug development and evaluation in this sector. In the meantime, the approaches outlined in this article serve as a guide for optimizing treat-ment of UTI from multidrug-resistant pathogens that currently have no available agents.

REFERENCES

1. Engemann JJ, Carmeli Y, Cosgrove SE, et al. Adverse clinical and economic outcomes attributable to methicillin resistance among patients with Staphylo-coccus aureus surgical site infection. Clin Infect Dis 2003;36(5):592–8.
2. Cosgrove SE, Kaye KS, Eliopoulous GM, et al. Health and economic outcomes of the emergence of third-generation cephalosporin resistance in Enterobacter species. Arch Intern Med 2002;162(2):185–90.
3. Stosor V, Peterson LR, Postelnick M, et al. Enterococcus faecium bacteremia: does vancomycin resistance make a difference? Arch Intern Med 1998; 158(5):522–7.
4. Cosgrove SE. The relationship between antimicrobial resistance and patient out-comes: mortality, length of hospital stay, and health care costs. Clin Infect Dis 2006;42(Suppl 2):S82–9.

5. Doi Y, Park YS, Rivera JI, et al. Community-associated extended-spectrum beta-lactamase-producing Escherichia coli infection in the United States. Clin Infect Dis 2013;56(5):641–8.

6. Huttner B, Jones M, Rubin MA, et al. Drugs of last resort? The use of polymyxins and tigecycline at US Veterans Affairs medical centers, 2005-2010. PLoS One 2012;7(5):e36649.

7. Gupta K, Scholes D, Stamm WE. Increasing prevalence of antimicrobial resistance among uropathogens causing acute uncomplicated cystitis in women. JAMA 1999;281(8):736–8.

8. Pitout JD, Church DL, Gregson DB, et al. Molecular epidemiology of CTX-M-producing Escherichia coli in the Calgary Health Region: emergence of CTX-M-15-producing isolates. Antimicrob Agents Chemother 2007;51(4):1281–6.

9. Pitout JD, Hanson ND, Church DL, et al. Population-based laboratory surveillance for Escherichia coli-producing extended-spectrum beta-lactamases: importance of community isolates with blaCTX-M genes. Clin Infect Dis 2004; 38(12):1736–41.

10. Pitout JD, Laupland KB. Extended-spectrum beta-lactamase-producing Enterobacteriaceae: an emerging public-health concern. Lancet Infect Dis 2008;8(3): 159–66.

11. Calbo E, Romani V, Xercavins M, et al. Risk factors for community-onset urinary tract infections due to Escherichia coli harbouring extended-spectrum beta-lactamases. J Antimicrob Chemother 2006;57(4):780–3.

12. Ho PL, Poon WW, Loke SL, et al. Community emergence of CTX-M type extended-spectrum beta-lactamases among urinary Escherichia coli from women. J Antimicrob Chemother 2007;60(1):140–4.

13. Ho PL, Wong RC, Yip KS, et al. Antimicrobial resistance in Escherichia coli outpatient urinary isolates from women: emerging multidrug resistance phenotypes. Diagn Microbiol Infect Dis 2007;59(4):439–45.

14. Lewis JS 2nd, Herrera M, Wickes B, et al. First report of the emergence of CTX-M-type extended-spectrum beta-lactamases (ESBLs) as the predominant ESBL isolated in a U.S. health care system. Antimicrob Agents Chemother 2007; 51(11):4015–21.

15. Rodriguez-Bano J, Navarro MD, Romero L, et al. Epidemiology and clinical features of infections caused by extended-spectrum beta-lactamase-producing Escherichia coli in nonhospitalized patients. J Clin Microbiol 2004;42(3): 1089–94.

16. Rodriguez-Bano J, Navarro MD, Romero L, et al. Bacteremia due to extended-spectrum beta -lactamase-producing Escherichia coli in the CTX-M era: a new clinical challenge. Clin Infect Dis 2006;43(11):1407–14.

17. Woodford N, Ward ME, Kaufmann ME, et al. Community and hospital spread of Escherichia coli producing CTX-M extended-spectrum beta-lactamases in the UK. J Antimicrob Chemother 2004;54(4):735–43.

18. Kang CI, Cheong HS, Chung DR, et al. Clinical features and outcome of community-onset bloodstream infections caused by extended-spectrum beta-lactamase-producing Escherichia coli. Eur J Clin Microbiol Infect Dis 2008; 27(1):85–8.

19. Vital signs: carbapenem-resistant Enterobacteriaceae. MMWR Morb Mortal Wkly Rep 2013;62(9):165–70.

20. Hidron AI, Edwards JR, Patel J, et al. NHSN annual update: antimicrobial-resistant pathogens associated with healthcare-associated infections: annual summary of data reported to the National Healthcare Safety Network at the

Centers for Disease Control and Prevention, 2006-2007. Infect Control Hosp Epidemiol 2008;29(11):996–1011.

21. Shepherd AK, Pottinger PS. Management of urinary tract infections in the era of increasing antimicrobial resistance. Med Clin North Am 2013;97(4):737–57.

22. Zhanel GG, Laing NM, Nichol KA, et al. Antibiotic activity against urinary tract infection (UTI) isolates of vancomycin-resistant enterococci (VRE): results from the 2002 North American Vancomycin Resistant Enterococci Susceptibility Study (NAVRESS). J Antimicrob Chemother 2003;52(3):382–8.

23. Swaminathan S, Alangaden GJ. Treatment of resistant enterococcal urinary tract infections. Curr Infect Dis Rep 2010;12(6):455–64.

24. Karki S, Land G, Aitchison S, et al. Long term carriage of vancomycin-resistant enterococci in patients discharged from hospital: a 12-year retrospective cohort study. J Clin Microbiol 2013;51(10):3374–9.

25. Mandell GL, Bennett JE, Dolin R. Mandell, Douglas, and Bennett's principles and practice of infectious diseases. 7th edition. Philadelphia: Churchill Livingstone/Elsevier; 2010.

26. Garau J. Other antimicrobials of interest in the era of extended-spectrum beta-lactamases: fosfomycin, nitrofurantoin and tigecycline. Clin Microbiol Infect 2008;14(Suppl 1):198–202.

27. Widerstrom M, Wistrom J, Ferry S, et al. Molecular epidemiology of Staphylococcus saprophyticus isolated from women with uncomplicated community-acquired urinary tract infection. J Clin Microbiol 2007;45(5):1561–4.

28. Chang S, Sievert DM, Hageman JC, et al. Infection with vancomycin-resistant Staphylococcus aureus containing the vanA resistance gene. N Engl J Med 2003;348(14):1342–7.

29. Beerepoot MA, den Heijer CD, Penders J, et al. Predictive value of Escherichia coli susceptibility in strains causing asymptomatic bacteriuria for women with recurrent symptomatic urinary tract infections receiving prophylaxis. Clin Microbiol Infect 2012;18(4):E84–90.

30. Foxman B. Editorial commentary: extended-spectrum beta-lactamase-producing Escherichia coli in the United States: time to rethink empirical treatment for suspected E. coli infections? Clin Infect Dis 2013;56(5):649–51.

31. Auer S, Wojna A, Hell M. Oral treatment options for ambulatory patients with urinary tract infections caused by extended-spectrum-beta-lactamase-producing Escherichia coli. Antimicrob Agents Chemother 2010;54(9):4006–8.

32. Falagas ME, Vouloumanou EK, Togias AG, et al. Fosfomycin versus other antibiotics for the treatment of cystitis: a meta-analysis of randomized controlled trials. J Antimicrob Chemother 2010;65(9):1862–77.

33. Oteo J, Bautista V, Lara N, et al. Parallel increase in community use of fosfomycin and resistance to fosfomycin in extended-spectrum beta-lactamase (ESBL)-producing Escherichia coli. J Antimicrob Chemother 2010;65(11): 2459–63.

34. Gupta K, Hooton TM, Naber KG, et al. International clinical practice guidelines for the treatment of acute uncomplicated cystitis and pyelonephritis in women: a 2010 update by the Infectious Diseases Society of America and the European Society for Microbiology and Infectious Diseases. Clin Infect Dis 2011;52(5): e103–20.

35. Prakash V, Lewis JS 2nd, Herrera ML, et al. Oral and parenteral therapeutic options for outpatient urinary infections caused by enterobacteriaceae producing CTX-M extended-spectrum beta-lactamases. Antimicrob Agents Chemother 2009;53(3):1278–80.

36. Ramphal R, Ambrose PG. Extended-spectrum beta-lactamases and clinical out-comes: current data. Clin Infect Dis 2006;42(Suppl 4):S164–72.

37. Keating GM, Perry CM. Ertapenem: a review of its use in the treatment of bac-terial infections. Drugs 2005;65(15):2151–78.

38. Curcio D. Treatment of recurrent urosepsis with tigecycline: a pharmacological perspective. J Clin Microbiol 2008;46(5):1892–3.

39. Korth-Bradley JM, Troy SM, Matschke K, et al. Tigecycline pharmacokinetics in subjects with various degrees of renal function. J Clin Pharmacol 2012;52(9): 1379–87.

40. Krueger WA, Kempf VA, Peiffer M, et al. Treatment with tigecycline of recurrent urosepsis caused by extended-spectrum-beta-lactamase-producing Escheri-chia coli. J Clin Microbiol 2008;46(2):817–20.

41. Satlin MJ, Kubin CJ, Blumenthal JS, et al. Comparative effectiveness of amino-glycosides, polymyxin B, and tigecycline for clearance of carbapenem-resistant Klebsiella pneumoniae from urine. Antimicrob Agents Chemother 2011;55(12): 5893–9.

42. Sandri AM, Landersdorfer CB, Jacob J, et al. Population pharmacokinetics of intravenous polymyxin B in critically ill patients: implications for selection of dosage regimens. Clin Infect Dis 2013;57(4):524–31.

43. Lee GC, Burgess DS. Treatment of Klebsiella pneumoniae carbapenemase (KPC) infections: a review of published case series and case reports. Ann Clin Microbiol Antimicrob 2012;11:32.

44. Daikos GL, Markogiannakis A. Carbapenemase-producing Klebsiella pneumo-niae: (when) might we still consider treating with carbapenems? Clin Microbiol Infect 2011;17(8):1135–41.

45. Warren JW, Abrutyn E, Hebel JR, et al. Guidelines for antimicrobial treatment of uncomplicated acute bacterial cystitis and acute pyelonephritis in women. Infectious Diseases Society of America (IDSA). Clin Infect Dis 1999;29(4): 745–58.

46. Patel SS, Balfour JA, Bryson HM. Fosfomycin tromethamine. A review of its anti-bacterial activity, pharmacokinetic properties and therapeutic efficacy as a single-dose oral treatment for acute uncomplicated lower urinary tract infec-tions. Drugs 1997;53(4):637–56.

47. Naber KG, Bartnicki A, Bischoff W, et al. Gatifloxacin 200 mg or 400 mg once daily is as effective as ciprofloxacin 500 mg twice daily for the treatment of pa-tients with acute pyelonephritis or complicated urinary tract infections. Int J Anti-microb Agents 2004;23(Suppl 1):S41–53.

48. Linden PK. Treatment options for vancomycin-resistant enterococcal infections. Drugs 2002;62(3):425–41.

49. Pogue JM, Paterson DL, Pasculle AW, et al. Determination of risk factors asso-ciated with isolation of linezolid-resistant strains of vancomycin-resistant Entero-coccus. Infect Control Hosp Epidemiol 2007;28(12):1382–8.

50. Eisenstein BI. Lipopeptides, focusing on daptomycin, for the treatment of Gram-positive infections. Expert Opin Investig Drugs 2004;13(9):1159–69.

51. Livermore DM, Mushtaq S. Activity of biapenem (RPX2003) combined with the boronate beta-lactamase inhibitor RPX7009 against carbapenem-resistant Enterobacteriaceae. J Antimicrob Chemother 2013;68(8):1825–31.

52. Endimiani A, Choudhary Y, Bonomo RA. In vitro activity of NXL104 in combina-tion with beta-lactams against Klebsiella pneumoniae isolates producing KPC carbapenemases. Antimicrob Agents Chemother 2009;53(8):3599–601.

53. Goldstein EJ, Citron DM, Tyrrell KL, et al. In vitro activity of Biapenem plus RPX7009, a carbapenem combined with a serine beta-lactamase inhibitor, against anaerobic bacteria. Antimicrob Agents Chemother 2013;57(6):2620–30.
54. Hirsch EB, Ledesma KR, Chang KT, et al. In vitro activity of MK-7655, a novel beta-lactamase inhibitor, in combination with imipenem against carbapenem-resistant Gram-negative bacteria. Antimicrob Agents Chemother 2012;56(7):3753–7.
55. Mushtaq S, Woodford N, Hope R, et al. Activity of BAL30072 alone or combined with beta-lactamase inhibitors or with meropenem against carbapenem-resistant Enterobacteriaceae and non-fermenters. J Antimicrob Chemother 2013;68(7):1601–8.
56. Ishii Y, Eto M, Mano Y, et al. In vitro potentiation of carbapenems with ME1071, a novel metallo-beta-lactamase inhibitor, against metallo-beta-lactamase- producing Pseudomonas aeruginosa clinical isolates. Antimicrob Agents Chemother 2010;54(9):3625–9.
57. Zhanel GG, Lawson CD, Adam H, et al. Ceftazidime-avibactam: a novel cephalosporin/beta-lactamase inhibitor combination. Drugs 2013;73(2):159–77.
58. Boucher HW, Talbot GH, Benjamin DK Jr, et al. 10 x '20 Progress–development of new drugs active against gram-negative bacilli: an update from the Infectious Diseases Society of America. Clin Infect Dis 2013;56(12):1685–94.
59. Perez F, Bonomo RA. Can we really use ss-lactam/ss-lactam inhibitor combinations for the treatment of infections caused by extended-spectrum ss-lactamase-producing bacteria? Clin Infect Dis 2012;54(2):175–7.
60. Bush K, Pucci MJ. New antimicrobial agents on the horizon. Biochem Pharmacol 2011;82(11):1528–39.

Diagnosis and Management of Fungal Urinary Tract Infection

Carol A. Kauffman, MD

KEYWORDS

- Candida • Fungal urinary tract infection • Fungus ball • Cystitis • Pyelonephritis
- Fluconazole • Amphotericin B • Flucytosine

KEY POINTS

- Most patients with candiduria are asymptomatic. Candidemia rarely results from asymptomatic candiduria.
- The most common risk factors for candiduria are increased age, female sex, antibiotic use, urinary drainage devices, prior surgical procedures, and diabetes mellitus.
- Treatment is indicated only for the following groups with asymptomatic candiduria: very low birth weight infants, patients undergoing urinary tract procedures, and neutropenic patients. The vast majority of patients should not be treated.
- Patients who have symptoms of urinary tract infection should be treated. The treatment of choice is oral fluconazole. Amphotericin B and fluctyosine are less desirable alternatives, and there is little role for amphotericin B bladder irrigation.
- Other antifungal agents, such as voriconazole, posaconazole, and the echinocandins, cannot be recommended for Candida urinary tract infections because very little active drug is found in the urine.

INTRODUCTION

When the terms funguria or fungal urinary tract infection are used, most physicians are referring to candiduria and urinary tract infections due to *Candida* species. Other fungi, including yeasts, such as *Cryptococcus neoformans* and *Trichosporon asahii*, and molds, such as *Aspergillus* species and members of the Mucorales, can involve the kidney during the course of disseminated infection, but rarely cause symptoms referable to the urinary tract.[1,2] Among the major dimorphic fungi, *Blastomyces dermatitidis* not uncommonly causes symptomatic prostatic infection, and both *B dermatitidis* and *Histoplasma capsulatum* can cause epididymo-orchitis, but typical urinary tract infections are not seen. *Candida* species appear to be unique in their ability to both colonize and cause invasive disease in the urinary tract.[3] This overview focuses only on candiduria and *Candida* urinary tract infection because they are common and many times present perplexing management issues.

Division of Infectious Diseases, Veterans Affairs Ann Arbor Healthcare System, University of Michigan Medical School, 2215 Fuller Road, Ann Arbor, MI 48105, USA
E-mail address: ckauff@umich.edu

Infect Dis Clin N Am 28 (2014) 61–74
http://dx.doi.org/10.1016/j.idc.2013.09.004
0891-5520/14/$ – see front matter Published by Elsevier Inc.

id.theclinics.com

EPIDEMIOLOGY

Candida species normally inhabit the gastrointestinal tract, the genital tract, and the skin of humans. Urine rarely yields *Candida* species in persons who do not have specific risk factors allowing the organism to gain ingress into and colonize the bladder mucosa. Hospitalized patients, especially those in the intensive care unit (ICU) acquire many risk factors during hospitalization, and candiduria is a common finding. A 1-day, point-prevalence survey of urine cultures obtained from hospitalized patients in hospitals throughout Europe found that *Candida* species were the third most common organism isolated from urine after *Escherichia coli* and *Enterococcus* species.[4]

A large multicenter surveillance study assessed 861 hospitalized patients with candiduria and found several very common risk factors, including urinary drainage devices in 83%, diabetes in 39%, and urinary tract abnormalities in 37%.[5] In an ICU setting, a multicenter study from Spain noted the following independent risk factors for candiduria: age older than 65 years, female sex, diabetes mellitus, prior antibiotics, mechanical ventilation, parenteral nutrition, and length of hospital stay.[6] Although studies are few, risk factors for candiduria for those in the community are similar to those in hospitalized patients, namely diabetes, indwelling urinary catheters, and antibiotics (**Box 1**).[7]

Although there often is concern that candiduria will lead to candidemia, this is uncommon in the absence of obstruction or urinary tract instrumentation. In the large prospective surveillance study noted previously, only 7 (1.3%) of 530 candiduric patients who were followed for 10 weeks developed candidemia.[5] Similarly, in an ICU setting from France, only 5 of 233 patients who had candiduria developed candidemia due to the same species 2 to 15 days later.[8] In another study from Brazil, comparison by genotyping of paired candiduric and candidemic isolates from individual patients showed no relationship in more than half of the patients.[9]

Several studies in ICU populations have reported that patients who have candiduria have increased mortality rates when compared with similar patients without candiduria.[6,8] In none of these studies was it shown that candiduria led to candidemia, which then caused the death of the patient. Others have documented the trend to increasing mortality in non-ICU hospitalized patients with candiduria[10,11] and have also reported that treatment had no effect on mortality rates.[10] It seems likely that candiduria is a marker for a seriously ill patient who requires indwelling devices for monitoring and treating underlying illnesses.

Box 1
Risk factors predisposing to candiduria[a]

- Older age
- Female sex
- Diabetes mellitus
- Antibiotic use
- Urinary tract obstruction
- Urinary tract surgery/instrumentation
- Urinary drainage device

[a] Most patients have several predisposing factors.

PATHOGENESIS

Candida species cause urinary tract infection by either the hematogenous or ascending routes. Most kidney infection occurs by hematogenous seeding during an episode of candidemia, but this event is usually asymptomatic with regard to urinary tract symptoms. Many studies in experimental animals have found that multiple microabscesses develop throughout the cortex after intravenous administration of *Candida albicans*.[12] The organisms penetrate through the glomeruli into the proximal tubules, and then are shed into the urine.[13] Most animals were able to clear *Candida* from the kidney within several weeks. Autopsy studies note renal cortical microabscesses in most patients who die with invasive candidiasis.[14]

The pathogenesis of ascending infection with *Candida* has not been studied in depth.[15] *Candida* strains found in the vagina are genetically related to the strains that cause candiduria in women with indwelling bladder catheters.[16] Presumably spread from the perineum into the bladder leads to colonization, and then retrograde spread occurs into the collecting system of the kidney.[12] The presence of an indwelling catheter allows for biofilm formation and persistence of the organism.[15] This has been shown for several species of *Candida*, but appears to be less likely with *Candida glabrata*.[12,17] Formation of fungus balls is a complication that leads to obstruction and great difficulty in eradicating the organism. The pathogenesis of fungus ball formation likely is tied to biofilm formation, allowing persistence of the organism.[15]

MICROBIOLOGICAL ASPECTS

There are no distinguishing characteristics of urinary tract infections because of the different *Candida* species. Most infections are due to *C albicans*; overall, this species accounts for 50% to 70% of isolates.[4–6,18] *C glabrata* is the second most common cause of urinary tract infections in most series,[18] but *Candida tropicalis* is the second most common species in some centers.[9,19] *Candida parapsilosis, Candida krusei,* and other unusual *Candida* species are less commonly found in urine (**Table 1**).

Certain types of patients have a higher risk of developing *C glabrata* urinary tract infection. These include patients with hematological malignancies and transplant recipients. In the largest prospective series of kidney transplant recipients who had *Candida* urinary tract infections, approximately 50% of all isolates were *C glabrata* and 30% were *C albicans*.[20] A study among hospitalized patients who had indwelling

Table 1	
Candida species causing candiduria and urinary tract infections	
Species	**Comments**
Candida albicans	Most common colonizing and infecting species (50%–70% in most series); most strains fluconazole susceptible
Candida glabrata	Second or third most common species (10%–35%, depends on geography); most common in older adults, uncommon in children; most strains fluconazole resistant
Candida tropicalis	Second or third most common species (10%–35%, depends on geography); most strains fluconazole susceptible
Candida parapsilosis	Uncommon in urine (1%–7%); common cause of central line–associated candidemia and neonatal candidiasis; most strains fluconazole susceptible
Candida krusei	Uncommon in urine (1%–2%); innately fluconazole resistant

bladder catheters found that independent risk factors for *C glabrata* candiduria were diabetes, ICU admission, and prior treatment with antibiotics and with fluconazole.[21] *C glabrata* has a distinct age distribution for both candidemia and urinary tract colonization and infection. It is most common in older adults and very uncommon in neonates and young children.[22,23]

DIAGNOSIS
General Principles

The most difficult task when faced with a patient with candiduria is deciding whether this finding represents a contaminated urine sample, an organism colonizing the bladder and/or catheter, or an infection of the upper or lower urinary tract. Additionally, candiduria may be a manifestation of candidemia rather than just a cardinal sign of a urinary tract infection. There are not sensitive diagnostic criteria available to help one sort through these different possibilities, and clinical judgment must be relied on in many circumstances.

Approach to the Patient With Candiduria

The initial task is to decide if the presence of candiduria represents contamination of the sample (**Box 2**).[24] It is wise to first repeat the culture, being certain that a clean-catch midstream urine has been obtained. If the second sample does not yield

---

Box 2
Approach to the patient with candiduria

- Asymptomatic patient
  - Repeat clean-catch urine culture to be sure not a contaminant
    - If cannot obtain clean-catch urine, obtain urine by catheterization
  - Candida grows on repeat culture: correct predisposing factors (stop antibiotics, remove catheter)
    - Repeat urine culture after correct predisposing factors
  - Culture remains positive: obtain ultrasound to look for obstruction
    - No obstruction: observe and do not treat
    - Obstruction present: urology consultation
      - Treat with fluconazole if procedure performed to correct obstruction
- Lower urinary tract symptoms: dysuria, frequency, urgency
  - Culture urine for bacteria: if present, treat with appropriate antibiotic
  - No bacteriuria or persistent symptoms after treatment with antibiotic: obtain ultrasound to look for obstruction and treat with fluconazole
    - Obstruction present: urology consultation
- Upper urinary tract symptoms: fever, flank pain
  - Culture urine for bacteria: if present, treat with appropriate antibiotic
  - No bacteriuria or persistent symptoms after treatment with antibiotic: obtain ultrasound to look for obstruction and treat with fluconazole
    - Obstruction present: urology consultation
    - Obtain blood cultures to look for candidemia

organisms, then candiduria reflected contamination only and no further workup need be done. If the patient is unable to perform a clean-catch midstream urine collection, sterile bladder catheterization should be performed to obtain a sample.

In patients who have candiduria and who have an indwelling urinary catheter, the catheter should be discontinued, if feasible, and then a second sample obtained several days later to see if the candiduria has disappeared. If so, no further studies need be done. In patients in whom a catheter is required, the catheter should be replaced and a urine sample collected through the new catheter. If candiduria disappears, the first sample merely reflected colonization and no further workup is needed.

Many patients will have persistent candiduria, and in these patients, the problem is to define whether they have bladder colonization, cystitis, or upper tract infection. Clinical manifestations sometimes can be useful in establishing whether the patient has a *Candida* urinary tract infection. Laboratory studies also are of some help, but there are overlapping findings in patients who have colonization with no need for treatment and those with a urinary tract infection who do need to be treated.

Clinical Manifestations

Most patients with candiduria are asymptomatic.[5] Hematogenous spread to the renal cortex is usually an asymptomatic event, although these patients usually have symptoms related to candidemia. Thus, fever, hypotension, and signs of sepsis can be found in these patients, but they do not have symptoms referable to the urinary tract. In these patients, diagnosis and treatment are aimed at the bloodstream infection, and the finding of candiduria is incidental.

Patients who have ascending *Candida* urinary tract infection have symptoms that are no different from those noted with bacterial infections. Patients with cystitis have urgency, frequency, dysuria, and suprapubic discomfort. Some will complain of pneumaturia, and a few may notice that they have passed particulate matter. Systemic symptoms and signs of infection are usually absent.

Patients who have *Candida* pyelonephritis usually manifest chills, fever, and flank pain.[25] Symptoms of lower tract infection, including dysuria and frequency, are frequently also present. Although some patients have an acute febrile illness, others do not appear acutely ill, but on imaging studies will be found to have upper tract involvement. Pyelonephritis is more often seen in diabetic patients, in older adults, and in women.

Severe, but uncommon, complications of pyelonephritis include emphysematous pyelonephritis, perinephric abscess, and papillary necrosis, all of which are associated with increased morbidity and usually require surgical intervention.[14] If a fungus ball, which is a mass of hyphae and yeast cells, forms in the collecting system, the patient may become oliguric and have increasing flank pain. Fungus balls that form in the bladder can remain asymptomatic until they cause obstruction of ureters and/or urethra.

Patients who have an indwelling bladder catheter do not have dysuria or frequency and usually complain of few symptoms,[26] and patients in the ICU often are unable to communicate about any symptoms that they might have. Both of these circumstances make differentiation of infection versus colonization especially difficult.

Laboratory Studies

Urinalysis and culture of urine are the obvious initial laboratory studies that should be performed. Unfortunately, neither provides much help in distinguishing colonization from infection. Pyuria is present in patients who have a *Candida* urinary tract infection. If the patient does not have an indwelling bladder catheter, pyuria is helpful in differentiating colonization from infection. However, pyuria is routinely found in patients who have an indwelling bladder catheter, so that it becomes a less useful clue to infection in this population. Unfortunately, candiduria occurs most often in patients with indwelling urinary catheters, and it is in these patients that the physician is most often faced with decisions about colonization versus infection.

Studies in the 1970s showed that quantitative cultures for *Candida*, in contrast to those for bacteria, did not separate into distinct zones defining infection and colonization.[24,27] Among patients without indwelling urinary catheters, kidney involvement was documented with urine colony counts from 10^4 to greater than 10^5 yeasts/mL. For patients who had indwelling catheters, colony counts in the same range (between 2×10^4 to >10^5 colony-forming units/mL) did not correlate with biopsy-proven kidney infection. In an experimental murine model in which *Candida* was given as an intravenous bolus, colony counts in the urine did not correlate with the number of organisms found in the kidney.[28]

The techniques routinely used in most clinical microbiology laboratories for the detection of bacteria are adequate for detecting yeasts in urine. However, *C glabrata* grows slowly, and the tiny colonies may not appear until after incubated for 48 hours. Almost all laboratories discard routine urine culture plates after 24 hours, and may well miss growth of *C glabrata*. The laboratory should be told that a *C glabrata* urinary tract infection is suspected and asked to hold the culture plates for 72 hours to look for slowly growing colonies. In addition, sending a urine sample for fungal culture, which routinely is held for several weeks, can be helpful.

Most clinical microbiology laboratories do not identify yeast isolates obtained from the urine to species level. This is both a cost-saving and time-saving measure based on the fact that most yeasts isolated from urine are only colonizers, which should not be treated. However, if a patient is thought to have a *Candida* urinary tract infection, knowledge of the species is crucial because many isolates of *C glabrata* and all isolates of *C krusei* are resistant to fluconazole, the standard treatment.

Antifungal susceptibility studies should be performed if *C glabrata* is isolated. In a minority of cases, the organism may be susceptible and fluconazole can be used; in many cases, however, the organism will be resistant, and other options will need to be explored. Most isolates of *C albicans, Candida parapsilosis*, and *Candida tropicalis* are susceptible to fluconazole, but resistance has been reported, and susceptibility testing should be sought for these species, as well as other unusual *Candida* species, if treatment is anticipated.

Other laboratory studies are not very helpful in defining whether a patient has a *Candida* urinary tract infection. Inflammatory markers are usually within normal limits; white blood cell count and percentage of neutrophils are not usually elevated. Serum creatinine is important to define kidney function and dosages of antifungal agents if treatment is needed.

Imaging Studies

Ultrasonography is the preferred initial study because of its simplicity and ready availability. It is valuable for documenting hydronephrosis, and in *Candida* pyelonephritis may show focal hypoechoic lesions in the kidney. Obstruction due to fungus balls at any level in the urinary tract can be delineated with ultrasonography.[23,29,30] It is essential to look for obstruction, as antifungal treatment is rarely successful if obstruction is not relieved.

Computed tomography urograms are helpful in demonstrating the cause of hydronephrosis, the presence of a perinephric abscess or fungus ball, and can evaluate the excretory function of the kidney (**Fig. 1**).

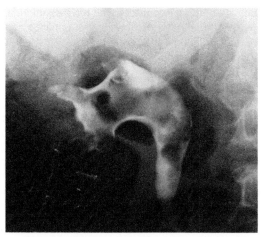

Fig. 1. Hydronephrosis and several fungus balls visualized as round masses excluding dye in excretory urogram of a patient with pyelonephritis due to *Candida albicans*.

TREATMENT
General Principles

Several concepts should be kept in mind when treating *Candida* urinary tract infections (**Box 3**). Asymptomatic candiduria should not be treated except in certain specific circumstances noted later in this article. Treatment must take into account the antifungal susceptibilities of the infecting species as well as the ability of the antifungal agent to achieve adequate concentrations in the urine. Fortunately, the most common species is *C albicans*, and most strains are susceptible to fluconazole, which is excreted into the urine as active drug.

The presence of indwelling urinary catheters makes eradication of candiduria very difficult. Often, simply removing the catheter without administering antifungal drugs and doing a follow-up urine culture will show that the host has been able to clear the organism from the urine.[5]

Equally important to remember is that if obstruction to urine flow is present anywhere in the genitourinary tract, antifungal agents will likely be ineffective in treating *Candida* urinary tract infection. Thus, an ultrasound study looking for obstruction should be done if the patient has persistent candiduria.

Box 3
General principles in the treatment of *Candida* urinary tract infections

- Asymptomatic candiduria should not be treated with antifungal agents, except in certain populations at risk for candidemia

- Antifungal susceptibilities and concentrations of antifungal agents in the urine are important factors in choosing the appropriate antifungal agent for *Candida* urinary tract infections

- Persistence of indwelling urinary catheters will likely prevent eradication of *Candida* with antifungal drugs

- Failure to relieve obstruction in the urinary tract will render antifungal therapy ineffective

Because bacteriuria is common in patients who have candiduria, treating the bacterial infection first is recommended. Many times the patient's symptoms clear with antibacterial therapy, and antifungal therapy is not needed. However, other patients require therapy for both bacteria and fungi to become asymptomatic.

Asymptomatic Candiduria

There are only a few circumstances in which asymptomatic candiduria should be treated (**Table 2**).[31,32] If a patient with candiduria is about to undergo a urological procedure, antifungal therapy should be given in the periprocedure period to prevent candidemia.[33,34] Asymptomatic candiduria also should be treated in patients who are neutropenic.[31] Symptoms may be minimal because of the neutropenia, and in this population, there is a high likelihood that candiduria reflects upper tract infection as a result of candidemia. Another patient population in which candiduria should always be treated is very low birth weight neonates. In these infants, candiduria is often a marker for invasive candidiasis and upper tract infection.[23,31]

Symptomatic Urinary Tract Infection

For patients who have persistent candiduria and symptoms of cystitis, treatment with oral fluconazole should be given (**Table 3**). The recommended dose is 400 mg initially, followed by 200 mg daily for 14 days based on the results of a multicenter, randomized, blinded, placebo-controlled trial.[31,35] Lower doses given for only a few days are discouraged, as Candida urinary tract infections should be viewed as complicated infections, requiring higher doses and longer treatment durations.

For patients who have persistent candiduria and whose symptoms suggest pyelonephritis, fluconazole is also the treatment of choice. The recommended dosage is 200 to 400 mg daily for 2 weeks.[31] Imaging of the urinary tract should be considered essential in any patient undergoing treatment for Candida pyelonephritis to evaluate for obstruction and the presence of complications, such as fungus ball formation, perinephric abscess, or emphysematous pyelonephritis.

Treatment of Complications

The most common complication is relapse of infection or failure to clear the infection after a course of fluconazole. If the patient has recurrent cystitis, imaging, urodynamic voiding studies, and cystoscopy should be performed. Prostatic abscess, bladder fungus ball, and chronic bladder changes due to long-standing infection all can contribute to relapse or failure to clear the infection. An extended course of fluconazole for susceptible organisms is indicated in these circumstances.

Table 2	
When to treat asymptomatic candiduria	
Patient Group	**Comments**
Patients undergoing a urological procedure	Risk of candidemia high following urinary tract instrumentation; treat with fluconazole immediately before and right after procedure
Neutropenic patients	High likelihood that candiduria represents candidemia with seeding to kidneys
Very low birth weight neonates	High likelihood that candiduria represents candidemia; high propensity to form renal fungus balls when candidemic

Table 3
Treatment of *Candida* urinary tract infections, with dosages for adult patients with normal kidney function

Indication	First-Line Treatment	Alternative Options for Resistant *Candida* Species
Asymptomatic candiduria in very low birth weight neonates or neutropenic patients	Treat for disseminated candidiasis: fluconazole, 400 mg qd × 2 wk	AmB, 0.5–1.0 mg/kg/d × 2 wk
Asymptomatic candiduria in patient about to undergo urological procedure	Fluconazole, 200–400 mg qd periprocedure	AmB, 0.3–0.6 mg/kg/d periprocedure
Cystitis	Fluconazole, 200 mg qd × 2 wk	AmB, 0.3–0.6 mg/kg/d × 1–7 d; 5-FC, 25 mg/kg tid × 7–10 d
Pyelonephritis	Fluconazole, 200–400 mg qd × 2 wk	AmB, 0.5–0.7 mg/kg/d × 2 wk; 5-FC, 25 mg/kg tid × 2 wk; or both AmB and 5-FC × 2 wk
Renal infection— hematogenous spread	Treat for disseminated candidiasis: fluconazole, 400 mg qd × 2 wk	AmB, 0.5–1.0 mg/kg/d × 2 wk
Fungus ball (bladder, ureter, or kidney)	Fluconazole, 200–400 mg qd until resolved; surgical removal	Local instillation of AmB an effective adjunct

Abbreviations: 5-FC, flucytosine; AmB, amphotericin B deoxycholate; qd, every day; tid, 3 times a day.

In patients who have upper tract *Candida* infection, obstruction is often found, and placement of a percutaneous nephrostomy tube or a ureteral stent may be required. This should be followed by a longer course of therapy with fluconazole, if the organism is susceptible.

The rare complications of emphysematous pyelonephritis and papillary necrosis almost always require nephrectomy. Drainage of a perinephric abscess is essential and is usually accomplished by interventional radiological techniques.

Patients in whom a fungus ball has been found should be treated with oral fluconazole and surgical or radiological interventions to relieve obstruction.[31] Nephrostomy tubes can be irrigated with amphotericin B deoxycholate to achieve high local concentrations. Given through this route, amphotericin B is not absorbed and is not nephrotoxic. Fluconazole also has been infused locally through nephrostomy tubes.[36] Local infusion is generally an interim procedure until the fungus ball can be removed by surgical or interventional radiological techniques.[37,38] It is imperative to maintain antifungal treatment when the fungus ball is being removed to prevent fungemia.

Special Problem of C glabrata Infection

C glabrata urinary tract infections, which are common in older adults, are often refractory to treatment. Removal of catheters, discontinuance of antibiotics, and relief of obstruction are essential. A higher dosage of fluconazole (800 mg daily) may provide adequate urine concentrations to eradicate this more azole-resistant organism. However, if the organism is totally resistant, then this approach will not succeed, and in patients with renal failure, the urine fluconazole concentrations may be too low to be effective.

An oral alternative is flucytosine, which is active against almost all strains of *C glabrata*.[31] Unfortunately, success rates are low, and adverse effects can be serious. Patients treated with this agent must be monitored carefully. Amphotericin B is probably the most effective agent, but requires placement of an intravenous catheter, and the drug's many side effects have to be dealt with.[31]

Echinocandins, which do not achieve adequate urine concentrations, have been tried; failure is the usual outcome, but success has been reported in a few cases.[39–42] Voriconazole and posaconazole, although active against *C glabrata*, do not achieve urine concentrations adequate to treat urinary tract infections. In some cases of recalcitrant cystitis, local irrigation of amphotericin B has been helpful in the short run, but definitive eradication remains elusive for many patients.

Antifungal Agents

Oral fluconazole is the agent of choice for treatment of *Candida* urinary tract infections.[31] It is effective for both upper and lower tract infections. Fluconazole achieves high urine levels, and most *Candida* species are susceptible to this agent. The exceptions are *C glabrata*, which is often fluconazole resistant, and *C krusei*, which is uniformly fluconazole resistant. The dosage of fluconazole should be reduced in patients who have reduced creatinine clearance (**Table 4**).

Fluconazole's urinary excretion is unique among azoles; all of the other azole agents, itraconazole, posaconazole, and voriconazole, are metabolized in the liver, and urinary excretion of active drug is either minimal or nil. As a result, none are recommended for treatment of *Candida* urinary tract infections.

Intravenous amphotericin B deoxycholate is effective in treating *Candida* urinary tract infections, but is generally reserved for instances in which fluconazole has proven to be ineffective. However, it is the treatment of choice for urinary tract infections caused by *C glabrata* or *C krusei*. The recommended dosage is 0.3 to 0.6 mg/kg per day for 5 to 7 days, but even single-dose treatment with 0.3 to 1.0 mg/kg has been shown to be effective.[43]

The lipid formulations of amphotericin B were introduced to reduce nephrotoxicity. It appears that they do not achieve adequate concentrations in the urine, and failures have been reported when these formulations have been used to treat *Candida* urinary

Table 4
Fluconazole and flucytosine dosing for *Candida* urinary tract infections in patients with reduced kidney function

Creatinine Clearance	Dosage
Fluconazole	
>50 mL/min	400 mg q 24 h
21–50 mL/min	200 mg q 24 h
<20 mL/min	200 mg q 48 h
Flucytosine	
>50 mL/min	25 mg/kg tid
21–50 mL/min	25 mg/kg bid
<20 mL/min	25 mg/kg qd

Abbreviations: bid, twice a day; q, every; qd, every day; tid, 3 times a day.

tract infections.[44] Thus, lipid formulations are not recommended for urinary tract infections.

Flucytosine has a limited but sometimes valuable role in treating fluconazole-resistant *C glabrata* urinary tract infections. This agent achieves high concentrations in the urine and is active against many isolates of *C glabrata*. *C krusei* is not susceptible to flucytosine. Flucytosine is often combined with amphotericin B. It can be used as a single agent, but resistance develops quickly.[31,32] Although the dosage recommended is 25 mg/kg 4 times daily for 7 to 10 days for cystitis and 14 days for upper tract infection,[31] this dosage is likely to cause bone marrow toxicity. For this reason, a lower dosage of 25 mg/kg 3 times daily is preferred. If there is renal dysfunction, the dosage should be decreased further (see **Table 4**).

None of the echinocandins are excreted into the urine as active drug, limiting their use for the treatment of urinary tract infections. However, there are reports of patients in whom caspofungin has been given to treat infection due to a fluconazole-resistant organism. Some reports note success and others document failure.[39–42] When these agents have been efficacious, it is generally in a patient in whom hematogenous dissemination to the kidney has occurred with candidemia. In these cases, it is possible that tissue concentrations in the kidney, rather than urine concentrations, are adequate and are most important for eradication.

Local Bladder Antifungal Infusion

Several trials have compared local bladder instillation of amphotericin B deoxycholate versus oral fluconazole for the treatment of candiduria.[45–47] Local instillation was effective in eliminating the organism from the bladder, but the effect was short-lived.

The usual daily dosage is 50 mg amphotericin B deoxycholate in 1 L sterile water, and instillation is done through an indwelling triple-lumen urinary catheter. An alternative method is the instillation of 100 mL of this solution several times daily through a regular indwelling catheter. The catheter is then clamped for 30 minutes, allowing the drug to remain in the bladder, and then unclamped.

Fluconazole bladder infusion has been used in patients with cystitis who have renal insufficiency and perhaps for that reason have failed oral fluconazole therapy.[48] The dose used was 200 mg in 1 L sterile saline daily.

Guidelines and commentaries on the management of urinary tract candidiasis do not recommend bladder instillation of antifungal agents,[31,49,50] but there are a few situations in which it can be helpful. For example, local infusion of amphotericin B can be used as adjunctive treatment for *C glabrata* or *C krusei* cystitis.

REFERENCES

1. Wise GJ, Talluri GS, Marella VK. Fungal infections of the genitourinary system: manifestations, diagnosis, and treatment. Urol Clin North Am 1999;26:701–18.
2. Kauffman CA. Fungal infections of the urinary tract. In: Schrier RW, Coffman TM, Falk RJ, et al, editors. Diseases of the kidney. 9th edition. Philadelphia: Lippincott, Williams, and Wilkins; 2013. p. 754–63.
3. Fisher JF. Candida urinary tract infections—epidemiology, pathogenesis, diagnosis, and treatment: executive summary. Clin Infect Dis 2011;52:S429–32.
4. Bouza E, San Juan R, Munoz P, et al. A European perspective on nosocomial urinary tract infections. I. Report on the microbiology workload, etiology, and antimicrobial susceptibility (ESGNI-003 study). Clin Microbiol Infect 2001;7:523–31.
5. Kauffman CA, Vazquez JA, Sobel JD, et al. Prospective multicenter surveillance study of funguria in hospitalized patients. Clin Infect Dis 2000;30:14–8.

6. Alvarez-Lerma F, Nolla-Salas J, Leon C, et al. Candiduria in critically ill patients admitted to intensive care medical units. Intensive Care Med 2003;29:1069–76.

7. Colodner R, Nuri Y, Chazan B, et al. Community-acquired and hospital-acquired candiduria: comparison of prevalence and clinical characteristics. Eur J Clin Microbiol Infect Dis 2008;27:301–5.

8. Bougnoux ME, Kac G, Aegerter P, et al. Candidemia and candiduria in critically ill patients admitted to intensive care units in France: incidence, molecular diversity, management, and outcome. Intensive Care Med 2008;34:292–9.

9. Binelli CA, Moretti ML, Assis RS, et al. Investigation of the possible association between nosocomial candiduria and candidemia. Clin Microbiol Infect 2006;12: 538–43.

10. Simpson C, Blitz S, Shafran SD. The effect of current management on morbidity and mortality in hospitalised adults with funguria. J Infect 2004;49:248–52.

11. Paul N, Mathai E, Abraham OC, et al. Factors associated with candiduria and related mortality. J Infect 2007;55:450–5.

12. Fisher JF, Kavenaugh K, Sobel JD, et al. *Candida* urinary tract infections—Pathogenesis. Clin Infect Dis 2011;52:S437–51.

13. MacCallum D, Odds F. Temporal events in the intravenous challenge model for experimental *Candida albicans* infections in female mice. Mycoses 2005;48: 151–61.

14. Kauffman CA. Candiduria. Clin Infect Dis 2005;41:S371–6.

15. Achkar JM, Fries BC. *Candida* infections of the genitourinary tract. Clin Microbiol Rev 2010;23:253–73.

16. Silva V, Hermosilla G, Abarca C. Nosocomial candiduria in women undergoing urinary catheterization. Clonal relationship between strains isolated from vaginal tract and urine. Med Mycol 2007;45:645–51.

17. Negri M, Silva S, Henriques M, et al. *Candida tropicalis* biofilms: artificial urine, urinary catheters, and flow model. Med Mycol 2011;49:739–47.

18. Sobel JD, Fisher JF, Kauffman CA, et al. *Candida* urinary tract infections—Epidemiology. Clin Infect Dis 2011;52:S433–6.

19. Kobayashi C, Fernandos O, Miranda C, et al. Candiduria in hospital patients: a prospective study. Mycopathologia 2004;158:49–52.

20. Safdar N, Slattery WR, Knasinski V, et al. Predictors and outcomes of candiduria in renal transplant recipients. Clin Infect Dis 2005;40:1413–21.

21. Harris AD, Castro J, Sheppard DC, et al. Risk factors for nosocomial candiduria due to *Candida glabrata* and *Candida albicans*. Clin Infect Dis 1999;29: 926–8.

22. Malani AN, Hmoud J, Chiu L, et al. *Candida glabrata* fungemia: experience in a tertiary care center. Clin Infect Dis 2005;41:975–81.

23. Phillips JR, Karlowicz MG. Prevalence of *Candida* species in hospital-acquired urinary tract infections in a neonatal intensive care unit. Pediatr Infect Dis J 1997;16:190–4.

24. Kauffman CA, Fisher JF, Sobel JD, et al. *Candida* urinary tract infections—Diagnosis. Clin Infect Dis 2011;52:S452–6.

25. Siddique MS, Gayed N, McGuire N, et al. Salient features of *Candida* pyelonephritis in adults. Infect Dis Clin Pract (Baltim Md) 1992;1:239–45.

26. Tambyah FS, Remmers AR, Perry JE. Catheter-associated urinary tract infection is rarely symptomatic: a prospective study of 1497 catheterized patients. Arch Intern Med 2000;160:678–82.

27. Sobel JD. Controversies in the diagnosis of candiduria: what is the critical colony count? Curr Treat Options Infect Dis 2002;4:81–3.

28. Navarro EE, Almario JS, Schaufele RL, et al. Quantitative urine cultures do not reliably detect renal candidiasis in rabbits. J Clin Microbiol 1997;35:3292–7.
29. Vasquez-Tsuji O, Campos-Rivera T, Ahumada-Mendoza H, et al. Renal ultrasonography and detection of pseudomycelium in urine as means of diagnosis of renal fungus balls in neonates. Mycopathologia 2005;159:331–7.
30. Kale H, Narlawar RS, Rathod K. Renal fungal ball: an unusual sonographic finding. J Clin Ultrasound 2002;30:178–80.
31. Pappas PG, Kauffman CA, Andes D, et al. Clinical practice guidelines for the management of candidiasis: 2009 update by the Infectious Diseases Society of America. Clin Infect Dis 2009;48:503–35.
32. Fisher JF, Sobel JD, Kauffman CA, et al. *Candida* urinary tract infections—Treatment. Clin Infect Dis 2011;52:S457–66.
33. Ang BS, Teklenti A, King B, et al. Candidemia from a urinary tract source: microbiological aspects and clinical significance. Clin Infect Dis 1993;17:662–6.
34. Gross M, Winkler H, Pitlik S, et al. Unexpected candidemia complicating ureteroscopy and urinary stenting. Eur J Clin Microbiol Infect Dis 1998;17:583–6.
35. Sobel JD, Kauffman CA, McKinsey D, et al. Candiduria: a randomized, double-blind study of treatment with fluconazole and placebo. Clin Infect Dis 2000;30:19–24.
36. Chung BH, Chang SY, Kim SI, et al. Successfully treated renal fungal ball with continuous irrigation of fluconazole. J Urol 2001;166:1835–6.
37. Bartone FF, Hurwitz RS, Rojas EL, et al. The role of percutaneous nephrostomy in the management of obstructing candidiasis of the urinary tract in infants. J Urol 1988;140:338–41.
38. Chitale SV, Shaida N, Burtt G, et al. Endoscopic management of renal candidiasis. J Endourol 2004;18:865–6.
39. Sobel JD, Bradshaw SK, Lipka CJ, et al. Caspofungin in the treatment of symptomatic candiduria. Clin Infect Dis 2007;44:e46–9.
40. Malani AN. Failure of caspofungin for treatment of *Candida glabrata* candiduria. Case report and review of the literature. Infect Dis Clin Pract (Baltim Md) 2010;18:271–2.
41. Schelenz S, Ross CN. Limitations of caspofugin in the treatment of obstructive pyelonephrosis due to *Candida glabrata* infection. BMC Infect Dis 2006;56:126–30.
42. Haruyama N, Masutani K, Tsuruya A, et al. *Candida glabrata* fungemia in a diabetic patient with neurogenic bladder: successful treatment with micafungin. Clin Nephrol 2006;66:214–7.
43. Fisher JF, Woeltke K, Espinel-Ingroff A, et al. Efficacy of a single intravenous dose of amphotericin B for *Candida* urinary tract infections: further favorable experience. Clin Microbiol Infect 2003;9:1024–7.
44. Augustin J, Raffalli J, Aguero-Rosenfeld M, et al. Failure of a lipid amphotericin B preparation to eradicate candiduria: preliminary findings based on three cases. Clin Infect Dis 1999;29:686–7.
45. Leu HS, Huang CT. Clearance of funguria with short-course antifungal regimens: a prospective, randomized, controlled study. Clin Infect Dis 1995;20:1152–7.
46. Jacobs LG, Skidmore EA, Freeman K, et al. Oral fluconazole compared with bladder irrigation with amphotericin B for treatment of fungal urinary tract infections in elderly patients. Clin Infect Dis 1996;22:30–5.
47. Fan-Havard P, O'Donovan C, Smith SM, et al. Oral fluconazole versus amphotericin B irrigation for treatment of candidal funguria. Clin Infect Dis 1995;21:960–5.

48. Marella VK, Ghitan M, Chapnock EK, et al. Fluconazole as an antifungal genito-urinary irrigant. Infect Dis Clin Pract (Baltim Md) 2006;14:158–60.

49. Sobel JD. Antifungal bladder irrigation. When and not how to treat candiduria? [editorial]. Infect Dis Clin Pract (Baltim Md) 2006;14:125–6.

50. Drew RH, Arthur RR, Perfect JR. Is it time to abandon the use of amphotericin B bladder irrigation? Clin Infect Dis 2005;40:1465–70.

Diagnosis and Management of Urinary Tract Infection in Older Adults

Theresa Anne Rowe, DO[a],*, Manisha Juthani-Mehta, MD[b]

KEYWORDS

- Aging • Elderly • Urinary tract infection • Asymptomatic bacteriuria

KEY POINTS

- Urinary tract infection (UTI) and asymptomatic bacteriuria (ASB) are common in older adults.
- Distinguishing UTI from ASB is problematic, as older adults may not present with typical signs and symptoms suggestive of UTI.
- Overutilization of antibiotics for suspected UTI is a major problem in older adults living in long-term care facilities, and leads to the development of multidrug-resistant organisms.
- Future studies to improve the diagnostic algorithm for UTI in older adults are needed.

DEFINITIONS OF URINARY TRACT INFECTION

Urinary tract infection (UTI) is one of the most commonly diagnosed infections in both hospitalized and community-dwelling older adults. The definition of symptomatic UTI in older adults generally requires the presence of localized genitourinary symptoms, urinary tract inflammation as demonstrated by pyuria, and a urine culture with an identified urinary pathogen (**Table 1**).[1] Although several consensus guidelines have developed UTI definitions for surveillance purposes, a universally accepted definition of symptomatic UTI in older adults does not exist.[1–4]

Funding Sources: Dr M. Juthani-Mehta: K23 AG028691, 1R01AG041153-01A1, Claude D. Pepper Older Americans Independence Center P30 AG021342; National Institute on Aging, National Institutes of Health; Dr T.A. Rowe: T32 AI007517-12.
Conflict of Interest: None.
[a] Yale University School of Medicine, 300 Cedar Street, New Haven, CT 06520-8002, USA;
[b] Section of Infectious Diseases, Department of Internal Medicine, Yale University School of Medicine, 300 Cedar Street, New Haven, CT 06520-8022, USA
* Corresponding author. Section of Geriatric Medicine, Department of Internal Medicine, Northwestern University School of Medicine, 750 N. Lake Shore Drive, Chicago, IL 60611.
E-mail address: theresa.rowe@northwestern.edu

Infect Dis Clin N Am 28 (2014) 75–89
http://dx.doi.org/10.1016/j.idc.2013.10.004
0891-5520/14/$ – see front matter

Table 1 Definition of common terms	
Pyuria	>10 white blood cells (WBC)/mm^3 per high-power field (HPF)
Bacteriuria	Urinary pathogen of $\geq$10^5 colony-forming units (cfu) per mL
Laboratory-confirmed UTI	Pyuria (>10 WBC/mm^3 per HPF) plus bacteriuria ($\geq$10^5 cfu/mL)
Asymptomatic bacteriuria	Bacteriuria in the absence of genitourinary signs or symptoms
Symptomatic UTI	Bacteriuria in the presence of genitourinary symptoms (ie, dysuria, suprapubic pain or tenderness, frequency, or urgency)
Uncomplicated UTI	Genitourinary symptoms (ie, dysuria, suprapubic pain or tenderness, frequency, or urgency) with evidence of pyuria plus bacteriuria in a structurally normal urinary tract
Complicated UTI	UTI occurring in a patient with a structural or functional urinary tract abnormality

DEFINITIONS OF ASYMPTOMATIC BACTERIURIA

Asymptomatic bacteriuria (ASB) is defined as the presence of bacteria in the urine in quantities of 10^5 colony-forming units per milliliter (cfu/mL) or more in 2 consecutive urine specimens in women or 1 urine specimen in men, in the absence of clinical signs or symptoms suggestive of a UTI.[5] Distinguishing UTI from ASB in older adults, although challenging, is particularly important, as antibiotics are necessary for the treatment of symptomatic UTI, but not for ASB. This review focuses on the most recent literature and guidelines on diagnosis, management, and prevention of both UTI and ASB in older adults.

EPIDEMIOLOGY OF URINARY TRACT INFECTION

Both ASB and UTI are common among older adults. UTI is the second most common infection diagnosed in the acute hospital setting,[6] and accounts for almost 5% of all emergency department visits by adults aged 65 years and older in the United States each year.[7] In long-term care facilities, UTI accounts for approximately 30% to 40% of all health care–associated infections, with an estimated point prevalence of 1.5% to 1.64%.[8,9] In community-dwelling older adults, the incidence and prevalence of UTI varies with age and gender. The incidence of UTI ranges from 0.07 per person-year in postmenopausal women[10] to 0.13 per person-year in adults older than 85.[11] The prevalence of UTI in one cohort study in women older than 65 years was found to be approximately 16.5% over a 6-month period.[12] Another cohort study in women older than 85 found almost 30% of women to have reported at least 1 UTI within a 12-month period.[13] In men, the annual incidence of UTI ranges from 0.05 in men aged 65 to 74 years and is estimated to increase to 0.08 in men aged 85 and older.[14] Although UTI is one of the most commonly reported infections in older adults, definitions for symptomatic UTI vary significantly across the literature, making the reported incidence and prevalence of symptomatic UTI in this population variable.

EPIDEMIOLOGY OF ASYMPTOMATIC BACTERIURIA

ASB is uncommon in younger adults, but increases significantly with age in both men and women. The prevalence of ASB is estimated to be between 6% and 10% in women older than 60 years and approximately 5% in men older than 65.[15] A cohort study by Rodhe and colleagues[16] found the prevalence of ASB in adults 80 years or older living in the community to be approximately 20% in women and 10% in men over an 18-month period. Almost 25% of individuals in this study with persistent ASB over 18 months had been treated with antibiotics, suggesting ongoing colonization despite antibiotic use. In institutionalized adults the incidence of bacteriuria is even higher, with estimates ranging from 25% to 50% for women and 15% to 35% for men.[15,17]

MICROBIOLOGY

Escherichia coli (*E. coli*) is the most frequent pathogen isolated from urinary cultures in both community-dwelling and institutionalized older adults.[12,18,19] Several population-based studies in community-dwelling postmenopausal women have found *E. coli* to be the most common urinary isolate, accounting for 75% to 82% of UTIs in this population. Other common organisms include *Klebsiella* spp., *Proteus* spp., and *Enterococcus* spp.[12,18] Organisms responsible for UTI and ASB in long-term care residents are similar to those in community populations. In a cohort of long-term care residents, *E. coli* was found to be the predominant organism, accounting for 53.6% of positive urine cultures. Other Enterobacteriaceae were also common and accounted for a total of 34.8% of cultures, specifically *Proteus* (14.6%), *Klebsiella* (13.9%), and *Providentia* (3.7%). Gram-positive organisms including *Enterococcus* and *Staphylococcus* accounted for 4.5% and 4.1% of cases, respectively.[19] Another larger study of older adults living in 32 long-term care facilities also found *E. coli* to be the most common organism isolated from urinary cultures, accounting for 69% of positive urine cultures in this cohort. *Klebsiella* spp. was the second most common (12%) followed by *Enterococcus faecalis* (8%).[20] It is postulated that the postmenopausal state, worsening incontinence and disability, and greater exposure to antibiotics changes the vaginal microbiome of older women, thereby changing the profile of uropathogens causing UTI in community-dwelling and institutionalized women. **Fig. 1** shows the most common organisms isolated from urine cultures in older adults.

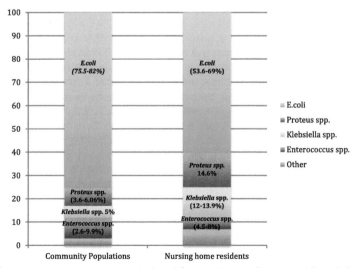

Fig. 1. The most common organisms isolated from urinary cultures in older adults.

ANTIMICROBIAL RESISTANCE

UTI is the most common reason for antimicrobial use in older adults, and inappropriate use of antibiotics leads to the development of multidrug-resistant organisms (MDROs). The high rate of ASB in older adults, particularly long-term care residents, often leads to overtreatment with antibiotics, and thus fosters the development of resistant pathogens in this population. A recent study in long-term care residents found a significant association between an increase in episodes of observed bacteriuria and isolation of multidrug resistant gram-negative rods.[21] Although MDROs are more common in health care settings, the prevalence of resistant urinary pathogens in community populations is also growing.[22] In a cohort of community-dwelling older women with UTI, 32% of *E. coli* urinary isolates were reported as resistant to trimethoprim/sulfamethoxazole (TMP/SMX), and 17% were resistant to fluoroquinolones. In women with ASB the rate of resistance was even higher, with 42% of urinary isolates reported as resistant to TMP/SMX and 35% resistant to flouroquinolones.[12] In a cohort of long-term care residents with bacteriuria, approximately 26% of all urinary isolates were found to be resistant to TMP/SMX and approximately 40% were resistant to fluoroquinolones. *E. coli*, in particular, had high rates of resistance to fluoroquinolones (60%), but was often sensitive to TMP/SMX (73%) and nitrofurantoin (93%).[19]

RISK FACTORS

A variety of factors predispose older adults to infections. Age-associated changes in adaptive and innate immunity may increase susceptibility to infections. Multiple medical comorbidities often increase the risk of hospitalization, in addition to the need for invasive procedures, prosthetic devices, and short-term and long-term urinary catheterization. Older adults are also more likely to reside in long-term care facilities, exposing them to nosocomial pathogens and increasing the risk of acquiring MDROs.[23]

Risk Factors in Older Community-Dwelling Older Adults

In community-dwelling older adults, one of the strongest predictors for developing UTI is having a history of UTI.[18,24] In a study of postmenopausal women aged 55 to 75 years, having a history of UTI increased the risk of UTI by more than 4-fold (odds ratio [OR] 4.20; 95% confidence interval [CI] 3.25–5.42) in comparison with postmenopausal women without a history of UTI.[25] Another study by Jackson and colleagues[10] found a significant increase in the risk of UTI in postmenopausal women with prior history of multiple UTIs. In this study, having a history of 6 or more UTIs increased the risk of having a subsequent UTI by almost 7-fold (hazard ratio [HR] 6.9; 95% CI 3.5–13.6). Other risk factors associated with developing UTI in older women include a history of urinary incontinence, presence of a cystocele, and a history of diabetes mellitus.[18,24] Sexual activity has also been associated with an increased risk of UTI in this population, although the association is not as strong as in premenopausal women.[18,26] A change in vaginal flora as a result of declining estrogen levels is thought to predispose postmenopausal women to UTI. However, oral estrogen replacement therapy has not been associated with prevention of UTI in this population.[18] In men, prostatic hypertrophy causing urinary retention and high postvoid residuals may be associated with developing UTI.[27] A recent study evaluating high postvoid residual in women did not find a significant association between women with postvoid residual of 200 mL or more and 1-year risk of developing a UTI when compared with women with postvoid residual of less than 50 mL, after adjustment for potential confounders.[28]

Risk Factors in Older Adults in Long-Term Care Facilities

Older adults residing in long-term care facilities are more likely to suffer from significant functional and cognitive impairments, both of which have been shown to increase the risk of developing UTI in this population. Disorders such as dementia, Parkinson's disease, and stroke often lead to voiding abnormalities, impede adequate self-hygiene, and increase the need for urinary catheterization. In a study by Eriksson and colleagues,[13] having a history of UTI within the previous year was significantly associated with vertebral fractures, multi-infarct dementia, and stroke. Many of these impairments have also been shown to increase the risk of persistent bacteriuria in older adults. In a cohort of long-term care residents without indwelling catheters, having persistent bacteriuria was significantly associated with requiring total nursing care, in comparison with adults with transient or no bacteriuria (OR 3.2; 95% CI 1.6–6.6). This study also concluded that persistent bacteriuria in women was significantly associated with the diagnosis of dementia (OR 2.4; 95% CI 1.2–4.8).[29]

DIAGNOSIS OF UTI IN COMMUNITY-DWELLING OLDER ADULTS

The diagnosis of symptomatic UTI in community-dwelling older adults who are cognitively intact requires the presence of genitourinary symptoms in the setting of urinary tract inflammation demonstrated by pyuria and a documented microbiologic pathogen. Symptoms suggestive of UTI in older adults are similar to those in younger patients, and include dysuria with or without frequency, urgency, suprapubic pain, or hematuria.[30] Older adults, however, may also initially present with generalized symptoms such as lower abdominal pain, back pain, and constipation.[25] Although urinary symptoms are common in community-dwelling older adults, not all patients who present with urinary symptoms have symptomatic UTI, and overuse of antibiotics for the treatment of UTI in this population remains a significant problem. A recent study by Little and colleagues[31] sought to examine the impact of several different management strategies on the use of antibiotics for cases of uncomplicated UTI in community-dwelling women. The investigators hypothesized that a delay in antibiotics would result in worse symptom control in comparison with immediate antibiotics. In this study, women suspected of having UTI were randomized into 1 of 5 different management approaches: (1) empiric immediate antibiotics, (2) delayed antibiotics (>48 hours), (3) antibiotics if 2 or more symptoms were present (cloudy urine, offensive urine odor, moderate to severe dysuria, or nocturia), (4) dipstick (antibiotics offered if nitrites or leukocytes and a trace of blood were detected), or (5) midstream urine (only symptomatic treatment until microbiology results were available). The investigators found no differences in symptom duration, severity of frequency symptoms, or severity of unwell symptoms between the antibiotic management strategies. However, they did find that use of urinary dipstick testing with a delayed prescription as backup, or empiric delayed prescriptions, helped to reduce antibiotic use. Almost all women in the immediate antibiotic group took antibiotics (97%), in contrast to those in the dipstick group (80%) and the delayed antibiotic group (77%). This study suggests that use of urinary dipstick with delayed antibiotic use may not lead to poorer symptom control and may reduce the use of antibiotics. The study included all women aged 18 to 70 years, so may not be applicable to older adults beyond the age of 70.[31]

Diagnostic Algorithm for UTI in Community-Dwelling Older Adults

In older adults who are cognitively intact and present with symptoms suggestive of UTI, a urinary dipstick to evaluate for the presence of nitrite or leukocyte esterase, along with a urinalysis, should be performed to evaluate for the presence of pyuria. Urinary culture is preferred to confirm the presence of bacteriuria and to evaluate for antimicrobial susceptibilities, although it is not required in all cases of uncomplicated UTI.[30] **Fig. 2** shows an algorithm proposed by the authors for use in community-dwelling older adults with suspected UTI.

DIAGNOSIS OF UTI IN LONG-TERM CARE FACILITIES

The diagnosis of symptomatic UTI in older adults residing in long-term care facilities is challenging, as most accepted definitions of UTI require the presence of localized genitourinary symptoms. Institutionalized older adults, however, often have significant underlying medical comorbidities such as dementia and stroke, which impair their ability to communicate, and are more likely present with atypical or nonspecific symptoms when infected.[1] Furthermore, older adults residing in long-term care facilities have a high prevalence of bacteriuria, making it difficult for providers to distinguish symptomatic UTI from ASB. In the past several decades, overtreatment of suspected UTI with antimicrobials has led to a variety of negative consequences, including the development of MDROs. To improve infection control practices and prevent the negative effects of overutilization of antibiotics, several consensus guidelines have been developed to assist providers in the diagnosis and treatment of UTI in long-term

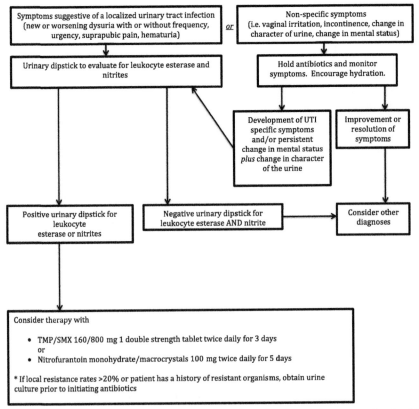

Fig. 2. Proposed diagnostic and empiric treatment algorithm for UTI in community-dwelling older adults.

care residents. In 1991, McGeer and colleagues[32] first proposed a set of infection definitions for surveillance purposes in long-term care facilities. According to the original McGeer criteria, the definition of symptomatic UTI for residents without an indwelling catheter includes at least 3 of the following signs and symptoms:

- Fever ($\geq$38°C) or chills
- New or increased burning pain on urination, frequency, or urgency
- New flank pain or suprapubic pain or tenderness
- Change in character of urine
- Worsening mental or functional status[32]

Although the original McGeer criteria were adopted for use by several regulating agencies, these criteria were never validated. In 2001, Loeb and colleagues[4] proposed a set of guidelines aimed to assist providers in prescribing antibiotics for residents in long-term care facilities. According to Loeb and colleagues, the minimum criteria for initiating antibiotics for UTI in residents without an indwelling urinary catheter include:

- Acute dysuria alone or
- Fever (>37.9°C or 1.5°C increase above baseline temperature) and at least 1 of the following:
- New or worsening
  - Urgency
  - Frequency
  - Suprapubic pain
  - Gross hematuria
  - Costovertebral tenderness
  - Urinary incontinence[4]

Although both the original McGeer and Loeb criteria are widely accepted, clinicians caring for patients in long-term care facilities often do not use them.[2,33,34] A recent study of 12 nursing homes in North Carolina found an overall low adherence to the Loeb criteria (0%–38.9%, mean 10.2%) when deciding on whether to institute antibiotic therapy for suspected UTI.[34] Furthermore, they did not find a significant association between adherence to the Loeb criteria and prescribing rates of antibiotics for UTI.

A significant challenge faced by clinicians when diagnosing symptomatic UTI in residents in long-term care facilities is the low incidence of localized genitourinary symptoms, many of which are necessary components of the original Loeb and McGeer criteria. In a recent study of long-term care residents with advanced dementia, the most common reason for suspected UTI was a change in mental status (44.3%). Localized genitourinary symptoms such as dysuria, urgency, and suprapubic pain were infrequent or absent.[33] In this study, almost 75% of residents who did not meet the minimum criteria for antibiotic initiation still received antibiotics.[33] Another study by Rotjanapan and colleagues[35] reported that more than 40% of patients living in 2 Rhode Island long-term care facilities who did not meet the original McGeer criteria for UTI still received antibiotics. These studies illustrate that although guidelines exist, providers often rely on components not included in the original McGeer or Loeb criteria, such as nonspecific symptoms, when deciding on whether to prescribe an antibiotic.

In 2007, a study of residents living in long-term care facilities in Connecticut attempted to identify features that would predict bacteriuria plus pyuria, both of which are necessary components in the diagnosis of UTI as they provide evidence of a host inflammatory response in the setting of a microbiological pathogen.

Dysuria, change in character of the urine (eg, gross hematuria, change in color of urine, change in odor of urine), and change in mental status (eg, change in level of consciousness, periods of altered perception, disorganized speech, or lethargy) were significantly associated with the outcome of bacteriuria plus pyuria. Dysuria alone predicted 39% of residents with bacteriuria plus pyuria; however, in combination with change in character of the urine or change in mental status, the predicted probability increased to 63%.[36] The positive predictive value for detecting bacteriuria plus pyuria using the original McGeer or Loeb criteria is 57%. These findings suggest that a combination of clinical features, which include change in mental status, should be further investigated and potentially incorporated into a diagnostic algorithm to be used by clinicians for diagnosing UTI. Although change in mental status is often reported by providers, only 3 measures of mental status (ie, periods of altered perception, disorganized speech, lethargy) and 1 measure of behavior (ie, resists care) have been shown to be reliably assessed by clinicians in nursing homes.[37] Falls, although a common reason for clinicians to suspect symptomatic UTI in nursing-home residents, have not been shown to be significantly associated with bacteriuria plus pyuria.[38]

In 2012 the Society for Healthcare Epidemiology of America (SHEA) updated the surveillance definitions of infections in long-term care facilities, based on the growing body of evidence-based literature on infections in older adults living in long-term care facilities.[3] These guidelines incorporated the acute care hospital surveillance definitions of the Centers for Disease Control and Prevention National Healthcare Safety Network. Major changes were made to the diagnosis of UTI for residents both with and without an indwelling urinary catheter. For residents without an indwelling urinary catheter, the diagnosis of UTI in the revised McGeer criteria includes:

Criteria from both 1 and 2
1. At least 1 of the following subcriteria of signs or symptoms
    - Acute dysuria or acute pain, swelling, or tenderness of the testes, epididymis, or prostate
    Or
    - Fever or leukocytosis and at least 1 of the following localizing urinary tract subcriteria
        - Acute costovertebral angle pain or tenderness
        - Suprapubic pain
        - Gross hematuria
        - New or marked increase in incontinence
        - New or marked increase in urgency
        - New or marked increase in frequency
    - In the absence of fever or leukocytosis, then 2 or more of the following localizing urinary tract subcriteria
        - Suprapubic pain
        - Gross hematuria
        - New or marked increase in incontinence
        - New or marked increase in urgency
        - New or marked increase in frequency
2. One of the following microbiological subcriteria
        - At least 10^5 cfu/mL of no more than 2 species of microorganisms in a voided urine sample
        - At least 10^2 of any number of organisms in a specimen collected by in-and-out catheter[3]

Diagnostic Algorithm for UTI in Older Adults in Long-Term Care Facilities

Although several guidelines are available to assist clinicians, diagnosing UTI in older adults remains challenging. According to the Infectious Disease Society of America (IDSA), the diagnostic laboratory evaluation of suspected UTI should be reserved for long-term care residents who present with acute onset of UTI-associated symptoms and signs (eg, fever, dysuria, gross hematuria, new or worsening urinary incontinence, and/or suspected bacteremia). The minimum laboratory evaluation for suspected UTI should include urinalysis to evaluate for pyuria and urinary dipstick to evaluate for evidence of leukocyte esterase and nitrite. If pyuria is present or the urinary dipstick is positive for leukocyte esterase or nitrite test, a urine culture should be obtained to evaluate for the presence of bacteriuria and to document antimicrobial susceptibility testing.[1] The absence of both leukocyte esterase and nitrite has been shown to have 100% negative predictive value for the diagnosis of UTI in long-term care residents suspected of having UTI.[39] In another study by Sundvall and Gunnarsson[40] evaluating 655 residents from 32 nursing homes, the negative predictive value for urinary dipstick was 88% for detecting bacteriuria. Thus, in most cases urinary culture should not be obtained in cases of a negative dipstick for leukocyte esterase and nitrite, and causes other than UTI should be evaluated. Urine culture alone often is not helpful in evaluating diffuse nonspecific symptoms in older long-term care residents[20] and should not be performed routinely in asymptomatic patients.[1] **Fig. 3** is a proposed algorithm based on the revised McGeer criteria, with additional suggestions by the authors based on adding empirically derived criteria.

MANAGEMENT

In older adults who present with nonspecific symptoms, identifying which patients require antibiotic treatment of symptomatic UTI is challenging. In the setting of uncertainty, clinicians frequently elect treatment with empiric antibiotics. This strategy, however, often leads to the overuse of antimicrobials and high rates of bacterial resistance. For most women who present with nonspecific symptoms, clinicians should encourage hydration and delay empiric antibiotic use until a diagnostic workup for UTI (ie, urinary dipstick, urine microscopy, urine culture) can be performed. A recent study by Knottnerus and colleagues[41] found that delaying antibiotics in women who present with nonspecific symptoms decreases the use of antibiotics. In this study, women who presented with symptoms suggestive of UTI were asked to delay antibiotic use. More than half of the women (55%) who delayed use had not used antibiotics after 1 week, and the majority (71%) of these patients reported improvement in their symptoms. None of the women who delayed antibiotics developed pyelonephritis.

In older adults with symptomatic UTI requiring antibiotics, selection of the optimal antimicrobial agent, dose, and duration should be chosen carefully to target the causative organism and minimize unwanted side effects. Older adults, particularly residents in long-term care facilities, often have baseline renal insufficiency, making it necessary to adjust common dosages using the estimated glomerular filtration rate.

Treatment of UTI in Community-Dwelling Older Adults

Treatment of uncomplicated UTI in older adults without significant medical comorbidities follows the same algorithm used in younger patients.[42] For treatment of uncomplicated UTI in women, the International Clinical Practice Guidelines proposed

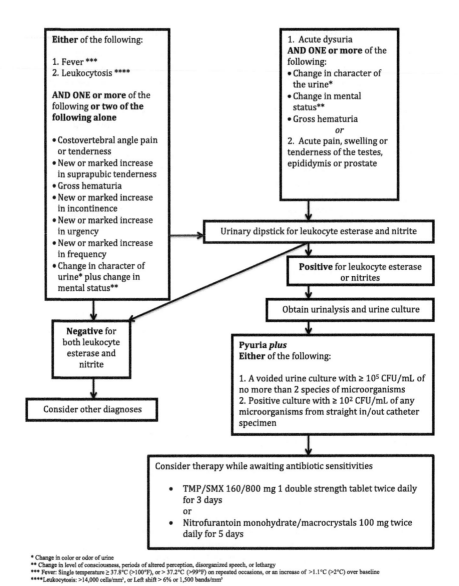

Either of the following:

1. Fever ***
2. Leukocytosis ****

AND ONE or more of the following or two of the following alone

• Costovertebral angle pain or tenderness
• New or marked increase in suprapubic tenderness
• Gross hematuria
• New or marked increase in incontinence
• New or marked increase in urgency
• New or marked increase in frequency
• Change in character of urine* plus change in mental status**

1. Acute dysuria
AND ONE or more of the following:
• Change in character of the urine*
• Change in mental status**
• Gross hematuria
   or
2. Acute pain, swelling or tenderness of the testes, epididymis or prostate

Urinary dipstick for leukocyte esterase and nitrite

Positive for leukocyte esterase or nitrites

Obtain urinalysis and urine culture

Negative for both leukocyte esterase and nitrite

Consider other diagnoses

Pyuria *plus*
Either of the following:

1. A voided urine culture with ≥ 10^5 CFU/mL of no more than 2 species of microorganisms
2. Positive culture with ≥ 10^2 CFU/mL of any microorganisms from straight in/out catheter specimen

Consider therapy while awaiting antibiotic sensitivities

• TMP/SMX 160/800 mg 1 double strength tablet twice daily for 3 days
   or
• Nitrofurantoin monohydrate/macrocrystals 100 mg twice daily for 5 days

* Change in color or odor of urine
** Change in level of consciousness, periods of altered perception, disorganized speech, or lethargy
*** Fever: Single temperature ≥ 37.8°C (>100°F), or > 37.2°C (>99°F) on repeated occasions, or an increase of >1.1°C (>2°C) over baseline
****Leukocytosis: >14,000 cells/mm³, or Left shift > 6% or 1,500 bands/mm³

Fig. 3. Proposed diagnostic algorithm for UTI in long-term care facilities for residents without an indwelling catheter.

by the European Society for Microbiology and Infectious Diseases and the IDSA recommend:

○ Nitrofurantoin monohydrate/macrocrystals, 100 mg twice daily for 5 days
Or
○ TMP/SMX, 160/800 mg, 1 double-strength tablet twice daily for 3 days

Fosfomycin (3 g as a single dose) is an acceptable alternative, although it may have inferior efficacy compared with other regimens. Antibiotics with local resistance rates greater than 20% should only be used if a urinary culture with antimicrobial sensitivity is available.[43] In men, the duration of antimicrobial treatment is often extended for a 7- to 14-day course. However, a recent study of UTI in male veterans found that longer duration of treatment (>7 days) was not associated with a reduction in the recurrence rate when compared with shorter-course treatment (<7 days), suggesting that shorter treatment in men may be warranted.[44] Further studies to evaluate the optimal treatment length of UTI in older men are needed.

Treatment of UTI in Older Adults in Long-Term Care Facilities

Both nitrofurantoin and TMP/SMX are acceptable empiric antimicrobial choices for residents in long-term care facilities. Nitrofurantoin is often underutilized in older adults because of its contraindication in patients with renal insufficiency. However, recent data suggest that nitrofurantoin is an effective agent for the treatment of UTI in older adults with a creatinine clearance greater than 40 mL/min.[45,46] Nitrofurantoin also has lower rates of overall resistance compared to TMP/SMX and fluoroquinolones, making it an effective empiric antibiotic choice for many older adults.[47] Although most *E. coli* isolates are susceptible to nitrofurantoin, other Enterobacteriaceae such as *Proteus mirabilis* may have intrinsic resistance to nitrofurantoin. In patients with a history of gram-negative infections with resistance to nitrofurantoin, TMP/SMX would be the preferred empiric antibiotic choice.[19] Residents of long-term care facilities, in whom treatment with antimicrobials for UTI is initiated, should have a urine culture obtained to test for antibiotic susceptibilities. Once available, antibiotics should be tailored based on antimicrobial susceptibility patterns. In most cases, the most narrow-spectrum antibiotic with activity against the confirmed microbiological pathogen should be used. In 2001, the SHEA recommended a 7-day course of antibiotics for women with a lower-level UTI residing in long-term care facilities; however, the optimal duration of antimicrobial treatment has not been well studied in this population.[48] For simple cystitis, a 3- to 5-day course of antibiotics is sufficient, as is used for younger populations.[43]

Treatment of ASB in Older Adults

Current guidelines do not recommend screening or treatment for ASB in older adults living in the community or living in long-term care facilities. Screening and treatment of ASB is only recommended in older adult men undergoing a urologic procedure in which mucosal bleeding is anticipated.[5]

PREVENTION

UTI is the most common reason antimicrobials are prescribed for older adults. Thus, prevention of UTI will lead to an overall decrease of antibiotic use in older adults. Several pharmacologic and nonpharmacologic strategies for prevention of UTI in older adults have been studied.

Mobility

Decreased mobility in aging adults has been shown to increase the risk for hospitalization for UTI. A recent retrospective cohort study by Rogers and colleagues[49] of older adults admitted to a long-term care facility found a significantly lower rate of hospitalization for UTI in patients who were able to walk. In this study, adults older than 65 years who were able to walk independently had a 69% reduction in risk of hospitalization for UTI in comparison with older adults who did not walk or required significant assistance. Residents who were able to maintain independent walking or show improvement in walking over time had a reduced risk of hospitalization for UTI by 53%

(HR 0.47, 95% CI 0.42–0.52). These results suggest that maintaining or improving mobility in older adults admitted to longer-term care facilities may protect against hospitalization for UTI.

Cranberry Formulations

Cranberry formulations have been used for the prevention and treatment of UTI for many years. Cranberry proanthocyanidin (PAC) is the active ingredient in cranberry that is thought to inhibit adherence of P-fimbriated *E. coli* to uroepithelial cells.[50] Although cranberry formulations have been used for the prevention of UTI, the efficacy of cranberry-containing products in preventing UTI is still unknown. In 1994 Avorn and colleagues[51] found a reduction in bacteriuria plus pyuria at 6 months in women living in long-term care and assisted living facilities who drank 10 ounces (300 mL) of cranberry-juice cocktail per day. This study concluded that 10 ounces of cranberry juice cocktail, which contained 36 mg of PAC, was effective in reducing bacteriuria and pyuria in this population. A recent Cochrane review, however, did not find significant evidence that ingestion of cranberry-containing products significantly prevented UTI, although there was a slight trend toward fewer UTIs in persons taking cranberry products.[52] A major limitation in many of the studies included in the Cochrane review is that many participants were unable to ingest the amount of cranberry juice with 36 mg of PAC that is necessary to show a potential benefit. The use of cranberry capsules containing 32 mg PAC has been shown to be a feasible alternative to cranberry juice in this population.[53] In a pilot study, the use of cranberry capsules containing 36 to 108 mg PAC found a trend toward a decrease in bacteriuria and pyuria in female nursing-home residents.[50] Future studies testing cranberry products with at least 36 mg PAC, preferably in capsule form, are needed to determine whether they are effective in preventing bacteriuria plus pyuria in older adults.

SUMMARY

The diagnosis of symptomatic UTI in older adults continues to be a significant challenge for providers caring for this population. Although guidelines are available to assist providers in diagnosing UTI, they are often not adhered to, and overtreatment with antibiotics remains an important issue. Future studies to improve the diagnostic criteria for UTI in older adults, particularly those living in long-term care facilities, are needed.

REFERENCES

1. High KP, Bradley SF, Gravenstein S, et al. Clinical practice guideline for the evaluation of fever and infection in older adult residents of long-term care facilities: 2008 update by the Infectious Diseases Society of America. Clin Infect Dis 2009; 48(2):149–71.
2. Juthani-Mehta M, Drickamer MA, Towle V, et al. Nursing home practitioner survey of diagnostic criteria for urinary tract infections. J Am Geriatr Soc 2005; 53(11):1986–90.
3. Stone ND, Ashraf MS, Calder J, et al. Surveillance definitions of infections in long-term care facilities: revisiting the McGeer criteria. Infect Control Hosp Epidemiol 2012;33(10):965–77.
4. Loeb M, Bentley DW, Bradley S, et al. Development of minimum criteria for the initiation of antibiotics in residents of long-term-care facilities: results of a consensus conference. Infect Control Hosp Epidemiol 2001;22(2):120–4.

5. Nicolle LE, Bradley S, Colgan R, et al. Infectious Diseases Society of America guidelines for the diagnosis and treatment of asymptomatic bacteriuria in adults. Clin Infect Dis 2005;40(5):643–54.
6. Curns AT, Holman RC, Sejvar JJ, et al. Infectious disease hospitalizations among older adults in the United States from 1990 through 2002. Arch Intern Med 2005;165(21):2514–20.
7. Caterino JM, Weed SG, Espinola JA, et al. National trends in emergency department antibiotic prescribing for elders with urinary tract infection, 1996-2005. Acad Emerg Med 2009;16(6):500–7.
8. Tsan L, Langberg R, Davis C, et al. Nursing home-associated infections in Department of Veterans Affairs community living centers. Am J Infect Control 2010;38(6):461–6.
9. Cotter M, Donlon S, Roche F, et al. Healthcare-associated infection in Irish long-term care facilities: results from the First National Prevalence Study. J Hosp Infect 2012;80(3):212–6.
10. Jackson SL, Boyko EJ, Scholes D, et al. Predictors of urinary tract infection after menopause: a prospective study. Am J Med 2004;117(12):903–11.
11. Caljouw MA, Den Elzen WP, Cools HJ, et al. Predictive factors of urinary tract infections among the oldest old in the general population. A population-based prospective follow-up study. BMC Med 2011;9:57.
12. Marques LP, Flores JT, Barros Junior Ode O, et al. Epidemiological and clinical aspects of urinary tract infection in community-dwelling elderly women. Braz J Infect Dis 2012;16(5):436–41.
13. Eriksson I, Gustafson Y, Fagerstrom L, et al. Prevalence and factors associated with urinary tract infections (UTIs) in very old women. Arch Gerontol Geriatr 2010;50(2):132–5.
14. Griebling TL. Urologic Diseases in America project: trends in resource use for urinary tract infections in men. J Urol 2005;173(4):1288–94.
15. Nicolle LE. Asymptomatic bacteriuria in the elderly. Infect Dis Clin North Am 1997;11(3):647–62.
16. Rodhe N, Lofgren S, Matussek A, et al. Asymptomatic bacteriuria in the elderly: high prevalence and high turnover of strains. Scand J Infect Dis 2008;40(10):804–10.
17. Hedin K, Petersson C, Wideback K, et al. Asymptomatic bacteriuria in a population of elderly in municipal institutional care. Scand J Prim Health Care 2002;20(3):166–8.
18. Hu KK, Boyko EJ, Scholes D, et al. Risk factors for urinary tract infections in postmenopausal women. Arch Intern Med 2004;164(9):989–93.
19. Das R, Perrelli E, Towle V, et al. Antimicrobial susceptibility of bacteria isolated from urine samples obtained from nursing home residents. Infect Control Hosp Epidemiol 2009;30(11):1116–9.
20. Sundvall PD, Ulleryd P, Gunnarsson RK. Urine culture doubtful in determining etiology of diffuse symptoms among elderly individuals: a cross-sectional study of 32 nursing homes. BMC Fam Pract 2011;12:36.
21. Das R, Towle V, Van Ness PH, et al. Adverse outcomes in nursing home residents with increased episodes of observed bacteriuria. Infect Control Hosp Epidemiol 2011;32(1):84–6.
22. Swami SK, Liesinger JT, Shah N, et al. Incidence of antibiotic-resistant *Escherichia coli* bacteriuria according to age and location of onset: a population-based study from Olmsted County, Minnesota. Mayo Clin Proc 2012;87(8):753–9.

23. Juthani-Mehta M, Quagliarello VJ. Infectious diseases in the nursing home setting: challenges and opportunities for clinical investigation. Clin Infect Dis 2010;51(8):931–6.
24. Raz R, Gennesin Y, Wasser J, et al. Recurrent urinary tract infections in post-menopausal women. Clin Infect Dis 2000;30(1):152–6.
25. Arinzon Z, Shabat S, Peisakh A, et al. Clinical presentation of urinary tract infection (UTI) differs with aging in women. Arch Gerontol Geriatr 2012;55(1):145–7.
26. Moore EE, Hawes SE, Scholes D, et al. Sexual intercourse and risk of symptomatic urinary tract infection in post-menopausal women. J Gen Intern Med 2008; 23(5):595–9.
27. Nicolle LE. Urinary tract infections in the elderly. Clin Geriatr Med 2009;25(3): 423–36.
28. Huang AJ, Brown JS, Boyko EJ, et al. Clinical significance of postvoid residual volume in older ambulatory women. J Am Geriatr Soc 2011;59(8):1452–8.
29. Eberle CM, Winsemius D, Garibaldi RA. Risk factors and consequences of bacteriuria in non-catheterized nursing home residents. J Gerontol 1993;48(6): M266–71.
30. Hooton TM. Clinical practice. Uncomplicated urinary tract infection. N Engl J Med 2012;366(11):1028–37.
31. Little P, Moore MV, Turner S, et al. Effectiveness of five different approaches in management of urinary tract infection: randomised controlled trial. BMJ 2010; 340:c199.
32. McGeer A, Campbell B, Emori TG, et al. Definitions of infection for surveillance in long-term care facilities. Am J Infect Control 1991;19(1):1–7.
33. D'agata E, Loeb MB, Mitchell SL. Challenges in assessing nursing home residents with advanced dementia for suspected urinary tract infections. J Am Geriatr Soc 2013;61(1):62–6.
34. Olsho LE, Bertrand RM, Edwards AS, et al. Does adherence to the Loeb minimum criteria reduce antibiotic prescribing rates in nursing homes? J Am Med Dir Assoc 2013;14(4):309.e1–7.
35. Rotjanapan P, Dosa D, Thomas KS. Potentially inappropriate treatment of urinary tract infections in two Rhode Island nursing homes. Arch Intern Med 2011; 171(5):438–43.
36. Juthani-Mehta M, Quagliarello V, Perrelli E, et al. Clinical features to identify urinary tract infection in nursing home residents: a cohort study. J Am Geriatr Soc 2009;57(6):963–70.
37. Juthani-Mehta M, Tinetti M, Perrelli E, et al. Interobserver variability in the assessment of clinical criteria for suspected urinary tract infection in nursing home residents. Infect Control Hosp Epidemiol 2008;29(5):446–9.
38. Rowe T, Towle V, Van Ness PH, et al. Lack of positive association between falls and bacteriuria plus pyuria in older nursing home residents. J Am Geriatr Soc 2013;61(4):653–4.
39. Juthani-Mehta M, Tinetti M, Perrelli E, et al. Role of dipstick testing in the evaluation of urinary tract infection in nursing home residents. Infect Control Hosp Epidemiol 2007;28(7):889–91.
40. Sundvall PD, Gunnarsson RK. Evaluation of dipstick analysis among elderly residents to detect bacteriuria: a cross-sectional study in 32 nursing homes. BMC Geriatr 2009;9:32.
41. Knottnerus BJ, Geerlings SE, Moll Van Charante EP, et al. Women with symptoms of uncomplicated urinary tract infection are often willing to delay antibiotic treatment: a prospective cohort study. BMC Fam Pract 2013;14:71.

42. Grover ML, Bracamonte JD, Kanodia AK, et al. Urinary tract infection in women over the age of 65: is age alone a marker of complication? J Am Board Fam Med 2009;22(3):266–71.
43. Gupta K, Hooton TM, Naber KG, et al. International clinical practice guidelines for the treatment of acute uncomplicated cystitis and pyelonephritis in women: a 2010 update by the Infectious Diseases Society of America and the European Society for Microbiology and Infectious Diseases. Clin Infect Dis 2011;52(5): e103–20.
44. Drekonja DM, Rector TS, Cutting A, et al. Urinary tract infection in male veterans: treatment patterns and outcomes. JAMA Intern Med 2013;173(1):62–8.
45. Oplinger M, Andrews CO. Nitrofurantoin contraindication in patients with a creatinine clearance below 60 mL/min: looking for the evidence. Ann Pharmacother 2013;47(1):106–11.
46. Bains A, Buna D, Hoag NA. A retrospective review assessing the efficacy and safety of nitrofurantoin in renal impairment. Can Pharm J 2009;142(5):248–52.
47. Mckinnell JA, Stollenwerk NS, Jung CW, et al. Nitrofurantoin compares favorably to recommended agents as empirical treatment of uncomplicated urinary tract infections in a decision and cost analysis. Mayo Clin Proc 2011;86(6):480–8.
48. Nicolle LE, SHEA Long-Term-Care-Committee. Urinary tract infections in long-term-care facilities. Infect Control Hosp Epidemiol 2001;22(3):167–75.
49. Rogers MA, Fries BE, Kaufman SR, et al. Mobility and other predictors of hospitalization for urinary tract infection: a retrospective cohort study. BMC Geriatr 2008;8:31.
50. Bianco L, Perrelli E, Towle V, et al. Pilot randomized controlled dosing study of cranberry capsules for reduction of bacteriuria plus pyuria in female nursing home residents. J Am Geriatr Soc 2012;60(6):1180–1.
51. Avorn J, Monane M, Gurwitz JH, et al. Reduction of bacteriuria and pyuria after ingestion of cranberry juice. JAMA 1994;271(10):751–4.
52. Jepson RG, Williams G, Craig JC. Cranberries for preventing urinary tract infections. Cochrane Database Syst Rev 2012;(10):CD001321.
53. Juthani-Mehta M, Perley L, Chen S, et al. Feasibility of cranberry capsule administration and clean-catch urine collection in long-term care residents. J Am Geriatr Soc 2010;58(10):2028–30.

Urinary Tract Infections in Special Populations

Diabetes, Renal Transplant, HIV Infection, and Spinal Cord Injury

Lindsay E. Nicolle, MD, FRCPC

KEYWORDS

- Urinary infection • Cystitis • Pyelonephritis • Asymptomatic bacteriuria • Diabetes
- Renal transplant • HIV infection • Spinal cord injury

KEY POINTS

- Patients with diabetes are more likely to present with complications of urinary infection, such as abscesses and emphysematous cystitis or pyelonephritis.
- Renal transplant patients have a high frequency of urinary infection because of multiple risk factors that may predate transplant, are associated with technical aspects of transplant surgery, or follow transplant.
- There is limited, if any, increased frequency of urinary tract infection directly attributable to HIV infection.
- Prevention of urinary tract infections in individuals with spinal cord injuries requires appropriate bladder management to maintain a low-pressure bladder, and avoidance of indwelling devices if possible.

INTRODUCTION

Some populations have unique considerations relevant to urinary tract infection. This article addresses 4 of these groups: patients with diabetes, patients with a renal transplant, patients with HIV infection, and patients with a spinal cord injury. Urinary tract infection occurring in these individuals is considered within the clinical category of complicated urinary infection; that is, infection that occurs in a patient with functional or structural abnormalities of the genitourinary tract. It is always important to distinguish between symptomatic urinary infection and asymptomatic infection, also referred to as bacteriuria, for optimal management of infection.

Health Sciences Centre, Room GG443, 820 Sherbrook Street, Winnipeg, Manitoba R3A 1R9, Canada
E-mail address: lnicolle@hsc.mb.ca

Infect Dis Clin N Am 28 (2014) 91–104
http://dx.doi.org/10.1016/j.idc.2013.09.006
0891-5520/14/$ – see front matter © 2014 Elsevier Inc. All rights reserved.

id.theclinics.com

PATIENTS WITH DIABETES
Unique Aspects of Urinary Infection

It is generally accepted that persons with diabetes have an increased frequency of urinary infection,[1,2] but there is limited evidence confirming the magnitude of excess risk.[3] In addition, the diabetic population is heterogeneous and the risk of urinary infection varies with patient characteristics. Several explanations have been proposed to explain an increased risk for infection, including glucosuria and impaired immune or leukocyte function,[2] but experimental studies have not consistently supported any single mechanism. The important diabetes-specific risk factors for urinary infection are usually duration of diabetes or presence of long-term complications, such as neuropathy, rather than current glucose control (**Table 1**).[4] There is limited evidence describing aspects of urinary infection in diabetic men. Of interest, the SGLT2 (serum glucose cotransporter-2) inhibitors, a new class of agents for treatment of diabetes that produce high levels of glucosuria, are associated with only a small increase in symptomatic urinary infection for both men and women.[7]

Epidemiology

Rates of urinary infection were compared between diabetic women enrolled in the epidemiology of diabetes interventions and complications study (Uro-EDIC) and nondiabetic women in the National Health and Nutrition Examination Survey III. The adjusted prevalence of cystitis in the preceding 12 months was similar (odds ratio [OR] 0.78; 95% confidence interval [CI]: 0.51, 1.22).[8] In the Uro-EDIC study, only sexual intercourse was associated with cystitis (OR 8.28; 95% CI 1.45, 158.32), similar to the nondiabetic population. Neither cystitis nor pyelonephritis was associated with duration of diabetes, hemoglobin A1c, retinopathy, neuropathy, nephropathy, vascular complications, or glycemic therapy. A prospective study from the Netherlands also reported that only sexual intercourse was associated with symptomatic infection in women with type 1 diabetes (relative risk [RR] 3.6; $P = .004$), whereas asymptomatic bacteriuria was the only significant association for type 2 diabetes (RR 1.65; 95% CI 1.02, 2.67).[5] Another prospective study enrolling women in a US health maintenance organization reported increased symptomatic urinary infection in postmenopausal women with diabetes (OR 2.2; 95% CI 1.6–3.0) for subjects receiving oral diabetes medication or insulin.[9] A retrospective record review of patients attending primary care practices in the Netherlands reported recurrent urinary infection was increased for women with diabetes (OR 2.0; 95% CI 1.4–2.9).[4] The increased risk was independently associated with type 2 diabetes, diabetes of 5 or more years' duration, receiving oral or insulin therapy, or retinopathy. Hemoglobin A1c was not a risk factor. Studies that have used administrative databases or retrospective record

Table 1		
Variables associated with symptomatic urinary tract infection or asymptomatic bacteriuria in women with Type 2 diabetes		
	Risk Factors for Infection (Ref.)	
	Symptomatic[4,5]	Asymptomatic[6]
Not diabetes associated	Age	Age
Diabetes associated	• Retinopathy • Oral hypoglycemic or insulin therapy • Diabetes ≥ 5 y	• Any long-term complication • Heart disease • Duration of diabetes • Oral hypoglycemic therapy

review, however, may overestimate the frequency of urinary infection in diabetic women, because these patients are more likely to seek medical care than nondiabetic persons.

Diabetes is a common risk factor associated with more severe presentations of urinary tract infection. A case series of 65 consecutive patients with renal or perinephric abscesses reported 28% of subjects had diabetes mellitus.[10] In other case series, 67% of patients presenting with emphysematous cystitis were diabetic,[11,12] and 62% presented with emphysematous pyelonephritis.[11] Diabetes mellitus has not, however, been identified as a risk factor for complications of severe sepsis or septic shock in patients with urosepsis.[13]

The prevalence of asymptomatic bacteriuria is increased for diabetic women but not diabetic men, with reported rates of 5% to 25% for women and 3% for men.[6] Asymptomatic bacteriuria correlates with duration of diabetes and long-term complications of diabetes, but not with parameters of current metabolic control (see **Table 1**).

Management

Diagnosis

The clinical and microbiologic diagnosis of urinary tract infection in diabetic populations is similar to other patients with complicated infection. Patients with neuropathy may have impaired bladder sensation, which obscures some clinical symptoms of lower tract infection. Diabetic women with pyelonephritis are more likely to have bilateral renal involvement and bacteremia. In a group of elderly Greek patients hospitalized with pyelonephritis, bacteremia was identified in 30.7% with and 11% without diabetes.[14] The types of infecting organisms are also similar for diabetic and nondiabetic patients.[15,16] *Escherichia coli* is the single most common organism. Strains isolated from women with or without diabetes have similar virulence characteristics.[3]

Treatment

Diabetic women with a functionally normal genitourinary tract are managed similarly to other women with uncomplicated urinary infection. Cystitis should be treated with short-course therapy and pyelonephritis for 7 to 14 days.[17] Complicated infections may require more prolonged antimicrobial therapy.[16] Imaging is indicated for severe clinical presentations, failure to respond to therapy, or early symptomatic recurrence following discontinuation of antimicrobial therapy. Emphysematous pyelonephritis is managed with antimicrobial therapy and initial percutaneous drainage; delayed nephrectomy, where necessary, is performed once the patient is stable.[11] A perinephric abscess usually requires percutaneous or open drainage. Small renal abscesses of less than 3 cm in diameter are treated conservatively with antimicrobial therapy alone and continued until the abscess has resolved on follow-up imaging.[10] This treatment may require prolonged therapy for several weeks to months.

Outcomes

Hospitalized elderly Greek diabetic patients with acute pyelonephritis had a longer duration of fever (median 4.5 vs 2.5 days, P<.001), a longer period of hospitalization (median 10 vs 7 days; P<.001), and higher mortality (12.5% vs 2.5% P<.01).[14] For women enrolled in 2 clinical trials evaluating ciprofloxacin therapy for treatment of acute uncomplicated pyelonephritis, diabetes mellitus was an independent predictor of treatment failure, defined as clinical failure or relapse by 4 to 6 weeks posttherapy (OR 8.3; 95% CI 2.3–30.3).[18] Diabetes is not, however, a reported risk factor for increased mortality for patients with septic shock from a urinary source.[12]

The contribution of symptomatic urinary infection to chronic kidney disease in patients with diabetes has been controversial. In 221 diabetic patients hospitalized from 2001 to 2011 for urinary infection complicated by systemic inflammatory response syndrome, evidence of acute kidney injury was present on admission only for subjects with preinfection glomerular filtration rate (GFR) of less than 30 mL/min.[19] In these patients, renal function had returned to baseline by 6 months following successful treatment of infection. The report describing elderly Greek patients with pyelonephritis also reported no significant association of diabetes with acute decline in renal function.[14]

Prevention

Women with frequent, recurrent cystitis and no evidence of impaired urinary function can be managed with long-term or postcoital antimicrobial prophylaxis strategies, similar to nondiabetic women.[15] Antimicrobial prophylaxis is not indicated for patients with impaired voiding attributable to neuropathy or with other genitourinary abnormalities, as prophylaxis does not decrease the subsequent frequency of symptomatic infection, whereas reinfection with antimicrobial-resistant organisms occurs. Underlying abnormalities should be corrected, if possible. Prevention of neuropathy should also prevent urinary tract infection for some patients. However, there are no studies of long-term diabetes management that specifically address the impact of prevention of long-term complications of diabetes on the frequency or severity of urinary infection. Treatment of asymptomatic bacteriuria in diabetic women does not decrease the frequency of symptomatic infection and, may, in the short term, increase episodes of infection including pyelonephritis.[20,21] Thus, asymptomatic bacteriuria should not be treated.

RENAL TRANSPLANT PATIENTS
Unique Aspects of Urinary Infection

Urinary tract infection is the most common infection occurring in renal transplant recipients.[22,23] Risk factors that promote urinary infection in these patients may predate transplant, be associated with the transplant procedure itself, or follow transplantation (**Table 2**). Patients with infection of native kidneys before transplant may have persistent infection following transplant because poor perfusion of the end-stage kidney limits antimicrobial access to the infection site and organisms cannot be eradicated. Technical aspects of the transplant procedure such as duration of use of an indwelling urethral catheter or ureteric stent increase the likelihood of infection. These indwelling devices become coated with biofilm, providing a persistent nidus for bacteriuria. Following transplantation, immunosuppressive therapy or persistent urologic abnormalities, such as strictures, stone formation, or hydronephrosis, increase the frequency of infection.

Epidemiology

From 25% to 47% of renal transplant patients experience at least one symptomatic urinary infection.[22,23] The risk of infection is highest in the first year following transplant. During a 10-year period from 1998 to 2008 a cohort of 122 Greek transplant patients experienced 316 episodes of urinary infection in 74 (60.7%) patients, with a mean follow-up of 67.8 months.[26] Asymptomatic bacteriuria and symptomatic episodes were not differentiated, but 141 episodes required hospitalization. Infection was diagnosed within 1 month posttransplant in 25% of all infected patients; 45% between 1 month and 1 year, 28% between the first and second year, and 48% after 2 years. There were 35 (29%) patients who experienced 3 or more infections. Urinary infection during the first month posttransplant correlated with recurrent urinary infection during any subsequent time period. Another single-center Polish study described

Table 2
Identified risk factors for increased frequency of urinary tract infection or bacteriuria following renal transplant

Exposure	Risk Factor
Pretransplant	Female
	Diabetes mellitus
	Prolonged dialysis
	Polycystic kidney disease
	Pretransplant urinary infection
Transplant procedure	Deceased donor
	Allograft trauma
	Microbial contamination of cadaver kidney
	Technical complications with anastomosis
	Indwelling urinary catheter
	Ureteral stent
Posttransplant	Urinary tract obstruction
	Immunosuppressive therapy
	Vesicoureteral reflux
	Reimplantation
	Acute rejection episodes

Data from Refs.[22,24,25]

the 12-month follow-up of all patients who received a transplant in 2009.[27] There were 151 episodes of urinary infection identified in 49 (55%) patients, with 48% diagnosed during the first month posttransplant. The clinical presentations were characterized as asymptomatic bacteriuria in 65%, lower urinary tract infection in 13%, and pyelonephritis in 22%.

Major risk factors for acute pyelonephritis following transplant are female gender (OR 5.14; 95% CI: 1.86, 14.20), experiencing acute rejection episodes (OR 3.84; 95% CI: 1.37, 10.79), number of urinary infections (OR 1.17; 95% CI: 1.06, 1.30), and receiving mycophenolate mofetil (OR 1.9; 95% CI: 1.2, 2.3).[24] In another report, identification of symptomatic or asymptomatic bacteriuria during the first year following transplant was independently associated with age (OR 1.04/year, 95% CI: 1.01, 1.07), female gender (OR 4.3; 95% CI: 2.01, 9.22), days of bladder catheterization posttransplant (OR 1.44/day; 95% CI: 1.05, 1.96), anatomic genitourinary alterations (OR 17.68; 95% CI 4.65, 67.29), and urinary infection during the month before transplantation (OR 4.98; 95% CI: 1.13, 21.96).[25]

Management

Diagnosis

The microbiological and clinical diagnosis of urinary tract infection is similar to other patients with complicated infection.[23,24] Graft tenderness is a clinical finding consistent with pyelonephritis in the transplanted kidney. A characteristic presentation is relapsing infection with a trimethoprim/sulfamethoxazole (TMP/SMX)-susceptible organism that presents after discontinuation of posttransplant TMP/SMX prophylaxis, suggesting persistent pretransplant infection in native kidneys, which was suppressed by the prophylactic therapy.

The appropriate quantitative count for asymptomatic or symptomatic infection is $\geq 10^5$ cfu/mL. Lower quantitative counts may be present for some symptomatic patients, such as patients undergoing diuresis. However, lower counts should be interpreted critically, particularly when ureteral stents are present, because biofilm formation on these devices may contaminate voided urine specimens. *E coli* remains the most common infecting organism. A wide spectrum of other organisms, including yeast, may be isolated depending on prior patient exposures and antimicrobial therapy.[22,24,27] These patients have frequent and prolonged exposure to health care settings and receive repeated courses of antimicrobials, so antimicrobial-resistant organisms are common.

Treatment

Treatment of symptomatic infection should, of course, avoid potential nephrotoxic agents. The selection of an antimicrobial regimen for empiric therapy must consider the likelihood that resistant organisms are present. Individuals developing urinary infection while receiving TMP/SMX will usually have a TMP/SMX-resistant organism isolated. Therapy in patients with renal impairment may need to be more prolonged, although the appropriate duration is not established. For patients who experience recurrent symptomatic infection, a systematic assessment should be undertaken to identify potentially contributing factors. Underlying urologic complications such as stones or strictures should be identified and corrected, if possible.

Prospective randomized clinical trials that address the question of treatment of asymptomatic bacteriuria for renal transplant patients have not been published. However, retrospective studies consistently report no benefits of treatment for preventing either symptomatic infection or poor graft outcomes.[28,29] In one report, 18.2% of treated patients and 5.6% of untreated patients with asymptomatic bacteriuria during the first posttransplant year had a composite outcome of hospitalization for symptomatic urinary infection or 25% reduction in estimated GFR.[29] Another report described 334 episodes of asymptomatic *E coli* or *Enterococcus faecalis* bacteriuria identified at least 1 month posttransplant in 77 patients at a Swiss center.[28] Symptomatic urinary infection developed following none of the treated episodes and in 1.7% of the untreated patients. These few symptomatic episodes were not complicated by either acute rejection or pyelonephritis. Spontaneous bacterial clearance was observed in 59% of untreated episodes. Recurrence followed 46% of treated episodes, and 78% of these recurrent episodes had more resistant strains isolated.

Outcomes

The prognosis of adequately treated symptomatic urinary tract infection is excellent. Transient decline of GFR may occur with acute pyelonephritis. However, symptomatic urinary tract infection is not a risk factor for impaired long-term graft function.[23,26,30]

Prevention

Identification and correction of urologic abnormalities will prevent further infections. Limiting the postoperative duration of an indwelling urethral catheter or ureteric stent decreases the risk for subsequent episodes of bacteriuria or symptomatic urinary tract infection.[31] A ureteric stent is usually placed routinely at surgery to assist with healing of the anastomosis. In a randomized controlled open-label study that compared ureteric stent removal at 8 or 15 days, asymptomatic or symptomatic urinary infection was significantly lower with early stent removal (40.5% vs 72.9%; *P* = .004).[31]

Renal transplant patients should receive TMP/SMX prophylaxis for 3 to 6 months following transplant,[32] decreasing the frequency of urinary tract infection as well as other infections. When recurrent symptomatic urinary infection is attributed to infection in native kidneys, prolonged suppressive antimicrobial therapy may be indicated to prevent symptomatic episodes. The antimicrobial regimen is selected based on tolerance and susceptibility of the infecting organisms and initiated at a full therapeutic dose. If this treatment is effective, the dose is decreased to one-half after 2 to 4 weeks.

There is no standard recommended duration of suppressive therapy. It may need to be continued for years for some patients.

Previously, recommendations suggested urine cultures should be collected routinely at follow-up visits, particularly for the first 6 months after transplant. Current guidelines do not recommend routine urine cultures for asymptomatic patients,[32,33] which reflects the increasing evidence that asymptomatic infection is not harmful and that treatment is not beneficial.

HIV INFECTION
Unique Aspects of Urinary Infection

The dominant immunologic abnormality of HIV infection is decreased cell-mediated immunity. Symptomatic uncomplicated urinary tract infection, on the other hand, correlates with variations of the innate immune response. It is unknown whether abnormalities of the innate immune system associated with HIV infection contribute to urinary tract infection, or how defects in cell-mediated immunity might promote urinary infection. Evidence is inconsistent in reporting whether there is an increased incidence of urinary tract infection directly attributable to HIV infection. In addition, there are few studies from the era of highly active antiretroviral therapy (HAART) therapy to characterize the current frequency of symptomatic urinary tract infection or bacteriuria in HIV-positive patients. Male patients with HIV infection may have an increased risk for prostatitis, but the contribution of HIV infection rather than other risk factors common in this population has not been determined.[34]

Epidemiology

The incidence of symptomatic urinary tract infection in a cohort of primarily male (89%) HIV patients followed between 1988 and 1992 was 1.49/100 patient-years overall, but 18.5/100 patient-years for women.[35] Patients with AIDS or a CD4 lymphocyte count less than 200 cells/mm^3 had an incidence of 5.4/100 patient-years compared with 0.5/100 for other HIV patients. In a prospective study of 1310 women, a self-reported history of urinary infection in the previous 6 months was significantly increased in women with HIV infection compared with matched seronegative at-risk women (OR 1.5; 95% CI 1.1–2.1), but infection did not correlate with CD4 cell count.[36] A subsequent report from the same cohort found no association of HIV infection with prevalence or incidence of asymptomatic bacteriuria.[37] HIV-infected women with bacteriuria had an increased viral load (RR 1.3; 95% CI 1.03–1.63), but not a lower CD4 count. In another report, symptomatic urinary infection occurred in 13.3% of men with a diagnosis of AIDS, 3.2% with asymptomatic HIV infection, and 1.8% without HIV infection.[38] However, the AIDS subjects in this report were hospitalized and the control groups were outpatients, so the comparison is subject to bias. An Internet-based survey addressing urinary quality-of-life outcomes for men reported that HIV infection was an independent risk factor for lower urinary tract symptoms consistent with prostatitis.[39] HIV-infected men had a worse total international prostate symptom score for all domains including quality of life, but the study did not differentiate between bacterial or nonbacterial prostatitis. A retrospective review of children aged 0 to 12 years who attended a South African clinic from 1996 to 2001 concluded that the clinical presentations, etiologic agents, response to therapy, and renal function of culture proven urinary tract infection were similar for HIV-infected or uninfected children.[40]

The prevalence of bacteriuria in Kenyan sex workers was reported to be 23% and was similar for women with or without HIV infection.[41] There was no correlation of bacteriuria with CD4 count for HIV-positive women. Of the 222 women enrolled,

19% reported lower tract symptoms or signs of fever and loin tenderness. There was no association between symptoms or signs of infection and HIV status. The prevalence of asymptomatic bacteriuria among pregnant HIV-positive women in Nigeria was 15.5%.[42] Bacteriuric women had significantly lower CD4 counts (250 cells/mm^3 vs 356/mm^3) and significantly higher viral loads (88,700 copies/mL vs 55,400 copies/mL). In another Nigerian study, 18% of HIV-positive pregnant women had asymptomatic bacteriuria.[43] Bacteriuria was independently associated with a past history of symptomatic urinary infection (OR 4.3; 95% CI 2.1, 7.9), HIV-1 RNA greater than 10,000 copies/mL (OR 3.9; 95% CI 2.7, 9.1), CD4 count less than 200 cells/mm^3 (OR 1.4; 95% CI 1.1, 3.3), and maternal hemoglobin less than 11 g/L (OR 1.4; 95% CI 1.3, 2.9). A cohort of HIV-infected men followed prospectively between 1987 and 1990 with urine cultures obtained every 6 months for 2 years identified bacteriuria in 30% of men with CD4 counts less than 200 cells/mm^3, 11% with 200 to 500 cells/mm^3, and in no subjects with cell counts greater than 500 cells/mm^3.[44]

Management

Clinical trials that address the diagnosis or therapy for urinary infection in HIV patients have not been reported. One review reported no significant difference in the frequency of symptomatic urinary tract infection for HIV patients receiving or not receiving TMP/SMX prophylaxis.[39] The frequency of symptomatic urinary tract infection identified in hospitalized Italian HIV patients (76% men) before and after the introduction of HAART was compared.[45] There were 5.6 episodes/100 person-years of urinary infection during the full period of observation. In a time series analysis, the proportion of patients with infection decreased from 9% to 4% (RR 1.94; 95% CI 1.5–2.5) after HAART became the standard of practice.[45] However, the authors did not stratify by potential sources of bias such as duration of hospitalization or indwelling catheter use, so the impact of HAART on frequency of urinary infection is uncertain.

SPINAL CORD INJURY
Unique Aspects of Infection

Spinal cord injury patients experience an increased frequency of urinary tract infection as a consequence of impaired bladder emptying associated with a neurogenic bladder.[46,47] Urinary tract infection and renal failure were the most common causes of death in these patients before the introduction of current bladder management strategies, which maintain a low-pressure bladder. A high bladder pressure leads to vesicoureteral reflux with hydronephrosis, pyelonephritis, and renal failure. Maintaining a low-pressure bladder in patients who cannot void spontaneously is usually achieved by intermittent catheterization or, for men, sphincterotomy and condom catheter drainage. Surgical procedures such as augmentation cystoplasty, ileal conduits, or other urinary diversions are also used for selected patients.[46] Some patients with high-level cord injury may require management with a chronic urethral or suprapubic urinary catheter.

Epidemiology

The incidence of symptomatic urinary infection in men with spinal cord injury is reported to be 0.41/100 person-days with intermittent catheterization and 0.36/100 person-days when a condom catheter is used.[48,49] This compares to 2.72/100 person/days with a chronic indwelling catheter. Risks for symptomatic infection include age greater than 40 years, hyperreflexic bladder with detrusor-sphincter dysynergy, a cervical level of injury, functional status, indwelling catheter, vesicoureteral reflux, and invasive procedure. The frequency and risks of infection are reported to be similar for men and women. Urinary infection is the most frequent cause of rehospitalization in the first year following traumatic spinal cord injury.

Asymptomatic bacteriuria is a common finding in spinal cord–injured patients with impaired voiding. The prevalence is 50% for patients with sphincterotomy or intermittent catheterization, and 100% with indwelling urethral or suprapubic catheters.[21] Risk factors for bacteriuria include detrusor sphincter dyssynergy, bladder overdistension, high-pressure voiding, large postvoid residual volume, urolithiasis, and vesicoureteral reflux. Quadriplegia, complete injury, and decreased functional independence are also associated with bacteriuria.[47]

Management

Diagnosis

Some patients will have a clinical presentation of increased lower limb hyperreflexia or increased incontinence associated with bladder spasms.[47] Individuals with high spinal cord lesions may present with autonomic dysreflexia. Clinical symptoms are, however, often nonspecific. Signs of urinary infection correlate poorly with urine cell counts and pyuria.[50] The accuracy and predictive value of signs and symptoms of urinary infection for asymptomatic or symptomatic infection were evaluated for patients using intermittent catheterization.[51] The highest accuracy for identification of a positive urine culture was cloudy urine (83.1%), and the highest specificity was fever (99%). However, fever had a very low sensitivity (6.9%). Subjects were able to predict a positive urine culture with an accuracy of 66.2%; the negative predictive value was 82.8% and positive predictive value was 32.6%. This study concluded that subjects were better at predicting the absence of urinary infection than a positive urine culture, when present.

The appropriate microbiologic quantitative criteria for diagnosis for spinal cord–injured patients using intermittent catheterization is $\geq 10^2$ cfu/mL of any organism, as these are catheterized specimens.[47] A wide variety of organisms are isolated, and resistant organisms are common.

Treatment

Antimicrobial selection is similar to other populations with complicated urinary tract infection.[47] In a prospective randomized trial, treatment of symptomatic urinary tract infection was less successful with 3 compared with 14 days of therapy.[52] Some patients experience frequent, recurrent infection with isolation of organisms of increasing antimicrobial resistance. In these patients, the recurrence should be characterized as relapse with the same organism, or reinfection with a new organism. Recurrent relapse following therapy for a susceptible organism suggests urolithiasis or, in men, prostate infection.

Prevention

The most important preventive strategy is to maintain a low-pressure bladder, with a bladder volume of less than 500 mL (**Box 1**).[46,48] Chronic indwelling urethral or suprapubic catheters should be avoided, if possible. Prophylactic antimicrobial therapy does not decrease the frequency of symptomatic infection and antimicrobial resistance emerges with reinfection, so prophylaxis is contraindicated.[48,53] Cranberry products are also not effective in preventing symptomatic infection.[54] In a multicenter study of patients enrolled in the early postinjury period, intermittent catheterization with a hydrophilic-coated catheter was not associated with a decreased incidence of symptomatic infection compared with a standard catheter.[55] However, a systematic review including all spinal cord injury populations concluded there was no difference in symptomatic urinary infection with hydrophilic-coated catheters compared

---

Box 1
Approaches to prevention of urinary infection in spinal cord injured subjects

Effective

- Maintain low-pressure bladder
  - Intermittent catheterization
  - Sphincterotomy/condom
  - Neobladder
- Intermittent catheterization
  - Education program (bacteriuria only)
- Avoid chronic indwelling catheter

Not effective

- Antimicrobial prophylaxis
- Cranberry products
- Hydrogel catheter

Investigational

- Bacterial interference
- Aerobic physical training

Data from D'Hondt F, Everaert K. Urinary tract infections in patients with spinal cord injuries. Curr Infect Dis Rep 2011;13:544–51; and Hooton TM, Bradley SF, Cardenas DD, et al. Diagnosis, prevention, and treatment of catheter associated urinary tract infection in adults: 2009 International Clinical Practice Guidelines from the Infectious Diseases Society of America. Clin Infect Dis 2010;50:625–63.

---

with uncoated catheters.[56] A prospective, randomized study compared standard care for management of patients with intermittent catheterization to an educational program of written material, self-administered test, and review by nurse and physician with follow-up telephone calls.[57] After controlling for baseline bacterial counts and differences between groups, patients randomized to the educational program had significantly fewer positive urine cultures, but no significant difference in symptom reports or antimicrobial treatment for urinary infection.

Treatment of asymptomatic bacteriuria does not decrease symptomatic infection and is associated with increased isolation of resistant organisms with reinfection.[52] Thus, treatment of asymptomatic bacteriuria is not indicated.[21,53] The optimal management of asymptomatic bacteriuria in pregnant women with spinal cord injury is not clear. Current guidelines recommend treatment of asymptomatic bacteriuria, similar to other pregnant women. However, recurrent bacteriuria is common, and resistant strains emerge requiring escalating courses of antimicrobial therapy. A small case series reported pregnant women with spinal cord injury were effectively managed with a weekly oral cyclic antibiotic program.[58] However, appropriate management of these women requires further evaluation.

Some innovative approaches for prevention have also been described. Bacterial interference is a strategy that induces asymptomatic bacteriuria using an avirulent *E coli* strain with a goal of preventing symptomatic infection with virulent strains. Preliminary studies report a small benefit of this intervention in decreasing symptomatic infection for selected spinal cord–injured patients.[59] In another novel approach, a randomized controlled trial of an aerobic physical training intervention reported a significant decrease in prevalence of chronic asymptomatic bacteriuria, but not symptomatic infection, in a small number of subjects. However, bladder management techniques for this study cohort were not characterized.[60]

REFERENCES

1. Hoepelman AI, Meiland R, Geerlings SE. Pathogenesis and management of bacterial urinary tract infections in adult patients with diabetes mellitus. Int J Antimicrob Agents 2003;22(Suppl 2):35–43.
2. Chen SL, Jackson SL, Boyko EJ. Diabetes mellitus and urinary tract infection: epidemiology, pathogenesis and proposed studies in animal models. J Urol 2009;182:S51–6.
3. Nicolle LE. Urinary tract infection in diabetes. Curr Opin Infect Dis 2005;18: 49–53.
4. Gorter KJ, Hak E, Zuithoff PA, et al. Risk of recurrent acute lower urinary tract infections and prescription patterns of antibiotics with and without diabetes in primary care. Fam Pract 2010;27:379–85.
5. Geerlings SE, Stolk RP, Camps MJ, et al. Risk factors for symptomatic urinary tract infection in women with diabetes. Diabetes Care 2000;23:1737–41.
6. Zhanel GG, Nicolle LE, Harding GK. Prevalence of asymptomatic bacteriuria and associated host factors in women with diabetes mellitus. Clin Infect Dis 1995;21:316–22.
7. Abdul-Ghani MA, Norton L, DeFronzo RA. Efficacy and safety of SGLT2 inhibitors in the treatment of Type 2 diabetes mellitus. Curr Diab Rep 2012;12:230–8.
8. Czaja CA, Rutledge BN, Cleary PA, et al. Urinary tract infections in women with type 1 diabetes mellitus: survey of female participants in the epidemiology of diabetes interventions and complications study cohort. J Urol 2009;181: 1129–35.
9. Boyko EJ, Fihn SD, Scholes D, et al. Diabetes and the risk of acute urinary tract infection among post-menopausal women. Diabetes Care 2002;25:1778–83.
10. Coelho RF, Schneider-Montero ED, Mesquita JL, et al. Renal and perinephric abscesses: analysis of 65 cases. World J Surg 2007;31:431–6.
11. Bjurlin MA, Hurley SD, Kim DY, et al. Clinical outcomes of nonoperative management in emphysematous urinary tract infections. Urology 2012;79:1281–5.
12. Thomas AA, Lane BR, Thomas AZ, et al. Emphysematous cystitis: a review of 135 cases. BJU Int 2007;100:17–20.
13. Nicolle LE. Urinary tract infection. Crit Care Clin 2013;29:699–715.
14. Kofteridis DP, Papademitraki E, Mantadakis E, et al. Effect of diabetes mellitus and the clinical and microbiological features of hospitalized elderly patients with acute pyelonephritis. J Am Geriatr Soc 2009;57:2125–8.
15. Nicolle LE. Uncomplicated urinary tract infection in adults including uncomplicated pyelonephritis. Urol Clin North Am 2008;35:1–12.
16. Durwood EN. Complicated urinary tract infections. Urol Clin North Am 2008;35: 13–22.
17. Gupta K, Hooton TM, Naber KG, et al. International clinical practice guidelines for the treatment of acute uncomplicated cystitis and pyelonephritis in women: a 2010 update by the Infectious Diseases Society of America and the European Society for Microbiology and Infectious Diseases. Clin Infect Dis 2011;52: e103–20.
18. Pertel PE, Haverstock D. Rick factors for a poor outcome after therapy for acute pyelonephritis. BJU Int 2006;98:141–7.

19. Chiu P-F, Huang C-H, Liou H-H, et al. Long term renal outcomes of episodic urinary tract infection in diabetic patients. J Diabet Complications 2013;27:41–3.
20. Harding GK, Zhanel GG, Nicolle LE, et al. Antimicrobial treatment in diabetic women with asymptomatic bacteriuria. N Engl J Med 2002;347:1576–83.
21. Nicolle LE, Bradley S, Colgan R, et al. Infectious Diseases Society of America guidelines for the diagnosis and treatment of asymptomatic bacteriuria in adults. Clin Infect Dis 2005;40:643–54.
22. Alangaden GJ. Urinary tract infections in renal transplant recipients. Curr Infect Dis Rep 2007;9:475–9.
23. Saemann M, Hoel WH. Urinary tract infection in renal transplant recipients. Eur J Clin Invest 2008;38(S2):58–65.
24. Rice JC, Safdar N. Urinary tract infections in solid organ transplant recipients. Am J Transplant 2009;9(S4):S267–72.
25. Sorto R, Irizar SS, Delgadillo G, et al. Risk factors for urinary tract infections during the first year after kidney transplantation. Transplant Proc 2010;42:280–1.
26. Papasotiriou M, Savvidaki E, Kalliakmani P, et al. Predisposing factors for the development of urinary tract infections in renal transplant recipients and the impact on the long-term graft function. Ren Fail 2011;33:404–10.
27. Golebiewska J, Debska-Slizien A, Komarnicka J, et al. Urinary tract infections in renal transplant recipients. Transplant Proc 2011;43:2985–90.
28. El Amari EB, Hadaya K, Buhler L, et al. Outcome of treated and untreated asymptomatic bacteriuria in renal transplant recipients. Nephrol Dial Transplant 2011;26:4109–14.
29. Green H, Rahaminov R, Goldberg E, et al. Consequences of treated versus untreated asymptomatic bacteriuria in the first year following kidney transplantation: retrospective observational study. Eur J Clin Microbiol Infect Dis 2013;32:127–31.
30. Fiorante S, Fernandez-Ruiz M, Lopez-Medrano F, et al. Acute graft pyelonephritis in renal transplant recipients: incidence, risk factors and long-term outcome. Nephrol Dial Transplant 2011;26:1065–73.
31. Parapiboon W, Ingsathit A, Disthabanchong S, et al. Impact of early ureteric stent removal and cost-benefit analysis in kidney transplant recipients: results of a randomized controlled study. Transplant Proc 2012;44:737–9.
32. Kasiske BL, Zeier MG, Chapman JR, et al. KD1G0 clinical practice for the care of kidney transplant recipients: a summary. Kidney Int 2010;77:299–311.
33. Kasiske BL, Vazquez MA, Harmon WE, et al. Recommendations for the outpatient surveillance of renal transplant recipients. J Am Soc Nephrol 2000;11:S1–86.
34. Shindel AW, Akhavan A, Sharlip ID. Urologic aspects of HIV infection. Med Clin North Am 2011;95:129–51.
35. Evans JK, McOwan A, Hillman RJ, et al. Incidence of symptomatic urinary tract infections in HIV seropositive patients and the use of cotrimoxazole as prophylaxis against Pneumocystits carinii pneumonia. Genitourin Med 1995;71:120–2.
36. Flanigan TP, Hogan JW, Smith D, et al. Self-reported bacterial infections among women with or at risk for human immunodeficiency virus infection. Clin Infect Dis 1999;29:608–12.
37. Park JC, Buono D, Smith DK, et al. Urinary tract infections in women with or at risk for human immunodeficiency virus infection. Am J Obstet Gynecol 2002;187:581–8.
38. De Pinho AM, Lopes GS, Ramos-Filho CF, et al. Urinary tract infection in men with AIDS. Genitourin Med 1994;70:30–4.

39. Breyer BN, Van den Eden SK, Horberg MA, et al. HIV status is an independent risk factor for reporting lower urinary tract symptoms. J Urol 2011;185:1710–5.
40. Asharam K, Bhimma R, Adhikari M. Human immunodeficiency virus and urinary tract infections in children. Ann Trop Paediatr 2003;23:273–7.
41. Ojoo J, Paul J, Batchelor B, et al. Bacteriuria in a cohort of predominantly HIV-1 seropositive female commercial sex workers in Nairobi, Kenya. J Infect 1996;33:33–7.
42. Awolude OA, Adesina OA, Oladokun A, et al. Asymptomatic bacteriuria among HIV positive pregnant women. Virulence 2010;1:130–3.
43. Ezechi OC, Gab-Okafor CV, Oladele DA, et al. Prevalence and risk factors of asymptomatic bacteriuria among pregnant Nigerians infected with HIV. J Matern Fetal Neonatal Med 2013;26:402–6.
44. Hopelman AIM, van Buren M, van den Brock J, et al. Bacteriuria in men infected with HIV-1 is related to their immune status (CD4 + cell count). AIDS 1992;6:179–84.
45. De Gaetano Donati R, Tumbarcello M, Tacconelli E, et al. Impact of highly active antiretroviral therapy (HAART) on the incidence of bacterial infections in HIV-infected subjects. J Chemother 2003;15:60–5.
46. Samson G, Cardenas DD. Neurogenic bladder in spinal cord injury. Phys Med Rehabil Clin N Am 2007;18:255–74.
47. D'Hondt F, Everaert K. Urinary tract infections in patients with spinal cord-injuries. Curr Infect Dis Rep 2011;13:544–51.
48. Hooton TM, Bradley SF, Cardenas DD, et al. Diagnosis, prevention, and treatment of catheter associated urinary tract infection in adults: 2009 International Clinical Practice Guidelines from the Infectious Diseases Society of America. Clin Infect Dis 2010;50:625–63.
49. Esclarin de Ruz A, Leoni EG, Cabrera RH. Epidemiology and risk factors for urinary tract infection in patients with spinal cord injury. J Urol 2000;164:1285–9.
50. Ronco E, Denys P, Bernede-Bauduin C, et al. Diagnostic criteria of urinary tract infection in male patients with spinal cord injury. Neurorehabil Neural Repair 2011;25:351–8.
51. Massa LM, Hoffman JM, Cardenas DD. Validity, accuracy and predictive value of urinary tract infection signs and symptoms in individuals with spinal cord injury on intermittent catheterization. J Spinal Cord Med 2009;32:568–73.
52. Dow G, Rao P, Harding G, et al. A prospective randomized trial of 3 or 14 days of ciprofloxacin treatment for acute urinary tract infection in patients with spinal cord injury. Clin Infect Dis 2004;39:658–64.
53. Everaert K, Lumen N, Kerckhaert W, et al. Urinary tract infections in spinal cord injury: Prevention and treatment guidelines. Acta Clin Belg 2009;64:335–40.
54. Opperman EA. Cranberry is not effective for the prevention or treatment of urinary tract infections in individuals with spinal cord injury. Spinal Cord 2010;48:451–6.
55. Cardenas DD, Morre KN, Dannels-McClure A, et al. Intermittent catheterization with a hydrophilic-coated catheter delays urinary tract infections in acute spinal cord injury: a prospective, randomized, multicenter trial. PM R 2011;3:408–17.
56. Bermingham SL, Hodgkinson S, Wright S, et al. Intermittent self catheterization with hydrophilic, gel reservoir, and non-coated catheters: a systematic review and cost effectiveness analysis. BMJ 2013;346:e8639.
57. Cardenas DD, Hoffman JM, Kelly E, et al. Impact of a urinary tract infection educational program in persons with spinal cord injury. J Spinal Cord Med 2004;27:47–54.

58. Salomon J, Schnitzler A, Ville Y, et al. Prevention of urinary tract infection in six spinal cord injured pregnant women who gave birth to seven children under a weekly oral cyclic antibiotic program. Int J Infect Dis 2009;13:399–402.
59. Darouiche RO, Hull RA. Bacterial interference for prevention of urinary tract infection. Clin Infect Dis 2012;55:1400–7.
60. Lavado EL, Cardoso JR, Silva LG, et al. Effectiveness of aerobic physical training for treatment of chronic asymptomatic bacteriuria in subjects with spinal cord injury: a randomized controlled trial. Clin Rehabil 2013;27:142–9.

Diagnosis, Management, and Prevention of Catheter-Associated Urinary Tract Infections

Carol E. Chenoweth, MD[a],*, Carolyn V. Gould, MD, MSCR[b], Sanjay Saint, MD, MPH[c]

KEYWORDS

- Prevention • Health care-associated • Urinary tract infection • ICU
- Urinary catheter

KEY POINTS

- Catheter-associated urinary tract infection (CAUTI) is often caused by hospital-based pathogens with a propensity toward antimicrobial resistance.
- The diagnosis of CAUTI is problematic because pyuria and bacteriuria are not reliable markers of infection. The treatment of bacteriuria in the absence of symptoms is not indicated, except in patients at risk of developing pyelonephritis or bloodstream infection (ie, pregnancy, urologic procedures with bleeding).
- Indwelling urinary catheters that have been in place for more than 2 weeks should be removed when treating CAUTI.
- The duration of urinary catheterization is the predominant risk for CAUTI; preventive measures directed at limiting the placement and early removal of urinary catheters significantly reduce CAUTI rates.
- Bladder bundles, collaboratives, and certain behaviors of hospital-based leaders are powerful tools for implementing preventive measures for CAUTI.

Disclosures/Conflict of Interest: C.E. Chenoweth, C.V. Gould: None; S. Saint: Honoraria and speaking fees from academic medical centers, hospitals, specialty societies, group-purchasing organizations (eg, Premier, VHA), state-based hospital associations, and nonprofit foundations (eg, Michigan Health and Hospital Association, Institute for Healthcare Improvement) for lectures about catheter-associated urinary tract infection and implementation science.
Disclaimer: The findings and conclusions in this report are those of the authors and do not necessarily represent the official position of the Centers for Disease Control and Prevention.
[a] Division of Infectious Diseases, Department of Internal Medicine, University of Michigan Health System, 3119 Taubman Center, 1500 East Medical Center Drive, Ann Arbor, MI 48109-5378, USA; [b] Centers for Disease Control and Prevention, 1600 Clifton Road Northeast, Mailstop A-31, Atlanta, GA 30333, USA; [c] Division of General Medicine, Department of Internal Medicine, University of Michigan Health System and Veterans Affairs Ann Arbor Healthcare System, 2800 Plymouth Road, Building 16, Room 430 West, Ann Arbor, MI 48109-2800, USA
* Corresponding author.
E-mail address: cchenow@umich.edu

Infect Dis Clin N Am 28 (2014) 105–119
http://dx.doi.org/10.1016/j.idc.2013.09.002
0891-5520/14/$ – see front matter
id.theclinics.com

Urinary tract infection (UTI) is one of the most common health care–associated infections (HAIs), representing up to 40% of all HAIs.[1–3] Most health care–associated UTIs (70%) are associated with urinary catheters, but as many as 95% of UTIs in intensive care units (ICUs) are associated with catheters.[4,5] Approximately 20% of patients have a urinary catheter placed at some time during their hospital stay,[6,7] especially in ICUs, in long-term care facilities, and increasingly in home care settings.[3,4,8] The Centers for Disease Control and Prevention (CDC) estimated that up to 139,000 catheter-associated UTIs (CAUTIs) occurred in US hospitals in 2007.[4]

CAUTIs are associated with increased morbidity, mortality, and costs. Hospital-associated bloodstream infection from a urinary source has a case fatality of 32.8%.[9,10] Each episode of CAUTI is estimated to cost $600; if associated with a bloodstream infection, costs increase to $2800.[11] Nationally, CAUTIs result in an estimated $131 million annual excess medical costs.[4]

Moreover, in October 2008, the Centers for Medicare and Medicaid Services (CMS) included hospital-acquired CAUTI under conditions that are no longer reimbursed for the extra costs of managing a patient.[11] To date, there has been no measurable effect of the CMS policy to reduce payments for CAUTIs on CAUTI rates or preventive practices.[12–14] Nevertheless, the prevention of CAUTIs has become a priority for most hospitals because 65% to 70% of CAUTIs may be preventable.[15]

EPIDEMIOLOGY OF CAUTIS

Likely as a result of widespread interventions occurring nationwide, rates of CAUTIs in ICUs reporting to the CDC decreased significantly between 1990 and 2007.[4] In 2010, the rates of CAUTIs reported to the CDC's National Healthcare Safety Network (NHSN) ranged from 4.7 per 1000 catheter-days in burn ICUs to 1.3 per 1000 catheter-days in medical/surgical ICUs.[4] Pediatric ICUs reported similar rates of CAUTI, 2.2 to 3.9 per 1000 catheter-days[16]; however, CAUTIs are infrequently identified in neonatal ICUs.[17] Inpatient wards reported rates equivalent to ICU settings, with a range from 0.2 to 3.2 per 1000 catheter-days. Among inpatient wards, rehabilitation units had the highest rates of CAUTIs.[5,16]

Microbial Cause of CAUTIs

Most microorganisms causing CAUTIs are from the endogenous microbiota of the perineum that ascend the urethra to the bladder along the external surface of the catheter.[18] A smaller proportion of microorganisms (34%) are introduced by intraluminal contamination of the collection system from exogenous sources, frequently resulting from cross-transmission of organisms from the hands of health care personnel.[18,19] Approximately 15% of episodes of health care–associated bacteriuria occur in clusters from patient-to-patient transmission within a hospital.[2,19] Rarely, organisms, such as Staphylococcus aureus, cause UTI from hematogenous spread.

Enterobacteriaceae, especially Escherichia coli and Klebsiella spp, are the most common pathogens associated with CAUTI; but in the ICU setting, Candida spp (18%), Enterococcus spp (10%), and Pseudomonas aeruginosa (9%) are more prevalent (**Table 1**).[16,20,21] European hospitals report a similar spectrum of microorganisms associated with nosocomial UTIs, except for Pseudomonas spp, which were isolated in only 7% of urine cultures.[22]

Among E coli isolates reported to the NHSN from CAUTIs in ICU and non-ICU settings in 2009 to 2010, 29.1% and 33.5%, respectively, were resistant to fluoroquinolones.[21] Many Enterobacteriaceae produced extended-spectrum beta-lactamases; 26.9% of K pneumonia/oxytoca and 12.3% of E coli isolates from patients with

Table 1		
Selected microorganisms associated with CAUTIs		
	LTACHs 2009–2010 % (Rank)	**NHSN All Units 2009–2010 % (Rank)**
Escherichia coli	14 (3)	26.8 (1)
Candida spp[a]	10 (5)	12.7 (3)
Enterococcus spp[a]	14 (3)	15.1 (2)
Pseudomonas aeruginosa	19 (1)	11.3 (4)
Klebsiella (pneumoniae/oxytoca)	17 (2)	11.2 (5)

Abbreviation: LTACH, long-term acute care hospitals.

[a] Species reported by Sievert et al[21] combined; therefore, rankings modified.

Data from Chitnis A, Edwards J, Ricks P, et al. Device-associated infection rates, device utilization, and antimicrobial resistance in long-term acute care hospitals reporting to the National Healthcare Safety Network, 2010. Infect Control Hosp Epidemiol 2012;33(10):993–1000; and Sievert D, Ricks P, Edwards J, et al. Antimicrobial-resistant pathogens associated with healthcare-associated infections: summary of data reported to the National Healthcare Safety Network at the Centers for Disease Control and Prevention, 2009–2010. Infect Control Hosp Epidemiol 2013;34(1):1–14.

CAUTIs were resistant to extended-spectrum cephalosporins. Alarmingly, during this same time period, 12.5% of Klebsiella spp from patients with CAUTIs were resistant to carbapenems.[21] Although long-term acute care hospitals (LTACHs) had a prevalence of carbapenem-resistant Enterobacteriaceae (CRE) in CAUTI isolates similar to that reported in ICUs, a greater percentage of LTACHs reported a CRE CAUTI compared with ICUs.[20]

Enterococci emerged as a commonly reported cause of health care–associated UTIs between 1975 and 1984. Although the clinical significance of enterococci isolated from urine is questionable, urinary drainage devices serve as a reservoir for emergence and spread of vancomycin-resistant strains in short- and long-term acute care settings.[20,21] Also rarely associated with complications when isolated from the urine,[23] Candida spp account for 28% of CAUTIs reported from ICUs.[20] S aureus are an infrequent cause of CAUTI but, when identified, should prompt consideration for coinciding bacteremia or endocarditis.[10,24] CAUTI associated with long-term catheters are associated with 2 or more organisms in 77% to 95% of episodes, and 10% have more than 5 species of organisms present.[3]

Biofilms, composed of clusters of microorganisms and extracellular matrix (primarily polysaccharide materials), form on the internal and external surfaces of urinary catheters shortly after insertion.[19,25] Typically, the biofilm is composed of one type of microorganism, although polymicrobial biofilms are possible. Microorganisms within the biofilm ascend the catheter to the bladder in 1 to 3 days. Antimicrobials penetrate into biofilms poorly, and microorganisms grow more slowly in biofilms, decreasing the effects of many antimicrobials.[19,25] The microorganisms, resistance patterns, and biofilm factors mentioned earlier have significant implications for the management of CAUTIs.

Risk Factors for CAUTIs

Table 2 outlines major modifiable and nonmodifiable risk factors for CAUTI, which have importance for the design and implementation of interventions for the prevention of CAUTI. The duration of catheterization is the dominant risk factor for CAUTI.[1,3,26] Women have a higher risk of UTI than men, and heavy bacterial colonization of the perineum increases that risk. Other factors that increase the risk of CAUTI include rapidly fatal underlying illness, more than 50 years of age, nonsurgical disease,

Table 2	
Risk factors for CAUTIs	
Modifiable Risk Factors	**Nonmodifiable Risk Factors**
Duration of catheterization	Female sex
Nonadherence to aseptic catheter care (ie, opening closed system)	Severe underlying illness
Lower professional training of inserter	Nonsurgical disease
Catheter insertion outside operating room	Aged >50 y Diabetes mellitus Serum creatinine >2 mg/dL

hospitalization on an orthopedic or urological service, catheter inserted outside the operating room, diabetes mellitus, and serum creatinine greater than 2 mg/dL at the time of catheterization. Nonadherence to aseptic catheter care recommendations has been associated with an increased risk of bacteriuria; conversely, systemic antibiotics have a protective effect on bacteriuria (relative risk 2.0–3.9).[2,3] Independent risk factors for urinary tract–related bloodstream infections in patients with bacteriuria include neutropenia, renal disease, and male sex.[27]

DIAGNOSIS OF CAUTIS

Clinical diagnosis of a CAUTI is challenging because pyuria and bacteriuria are almost uniformly present, but neither are reliable indicators of symptomatic UTI in the setting of catheterization.[28–31] Symptomatic UTI is defined by the presence of symptoms or signs referable to the urinary tract associated with significant bacteriuria.[28] Fever or other systemic symptoms may be the only clinical indication of UTI in patients who are critically ill or who have spinal cord injuries.[2,3] However, outside these patient populations, additional urinary tract-specific signs and symptoms should be sought for the diagnosis of UTI.[28,30]

Defining significant bacteriuria is difficult because some level of bacterial colonization is universal in urine from catheterized patients. Colony counts in urine as low as 10^2 colony-forming units (CFU)/mL can be associated with symptoms, and colony counts of this level rapidly increase to more than 10^5 CFU/mL within 24 to 48 hours.[28,32,33] Therefore, the National Institute on Disability and Rehabilitative Research defined bacteriuria in catheterized patients as growth of 10^2 CFU/mL or more of a predominant microorganism.[33] Other guidelines have defined 10^3 CFU/mL as a more reasonable threshold for significant bacteriuria, balancing the sensitivity of detecting CAUTI with the feasibility of the microbiology laboratory to quantify microorganisms.[28]

Asymptomatic bacteriuria is defined as bacteriuria in patients without signs or symptoms referable to the urinary tract.[28] The distinction from symptomatic UTI is clinically important because asymptomatic catheter-associated bacteriuria and funguria rarely result in adverse outcomes (eg, pyelonephritis, perinephric abscess, bacteremia) and generally do not require treatment.[30] Nevertheless, a large proportion of antimicrobials in hospitalized patients are prescribed for the treatment of UTIs, most often asymptomatic bacteriuria.[34–36]

MANAGEMENT OF CAUTIS

The treatment of asymptomatic catheter-associated bacteriuria or candiduria is not indicated except in patients who are at a high risk for the development of complications, such as pyelonephritis or bloodstream infection.[37] Screening and treating pregnant women for asymptomatic bacteriuria to prevent pyelonephritis are recommended. In addition, patients undergoing genitourinary procedures likely to induce mucosal bleeding should be screened and treated in advance for asymptomatic bacteriuria.[28,37] As with asymptomatic bacteriuria, asymptomatic candiduria generally does not require treatment, except in neutropenic patients and other high-risk patients noted earlier.[38] Furthermore, because of poor specificity of fever and frequency of bacteriuria and funguria in hospitalized patients with urinary catheters, a thorough investigation for other sources of fever should be conducted before diagnosing a UTI.

Asymptomatic bacteriuria, persisting for 48 hours after the removal of a urinary catheter, has a high risk of progressing to symptomatic UTI; treatment in hospitalized women has been shown to decrease the risk of subsequent UTIs.[39] Therefore, considering the treatment of women with asymptomatic bacteriuria persisting 48 hours after catheter removal is recommended.[28,37,39] When indicated, 3 to 7 days of appropriate antimicrobial therapy based on culture results should be adequate for the treatment of asymptomatic bacteriuria.[28,37]

Repeated antimicrobial treatment of bacteriuria during long-term catheterization is a significant risk for colonization with multidrug-resistant organisms, and most of this use is inappropriate.[34,35] A recent study reported that a 1-hour educational session reduced inappropriate use of antibiotic therapy for inpatients with positive urine cultures.[40] In addition, audit and feedback to care providers decreased overdiagnosis of CAUTIs and associated inappropriate antibiotic use in another study.[36] Educational efforts aimed at reducing unnecessary urine cultures (eg, pan-culturing for fever without a thorough clinical assessment) would also prevent the inappropriate treatment of bacteriuria and funguria.

Because of the presence of biofilm, leaving the catheter in place during the treatment of CAUTIs makes eradicating bacteriuria or candiduria difficult and can lead to the development of antimicrobial resistance. The management of symptomatic CAUTIs should include removing or replacing the urinary catheter if it has been in place for at least 2 weeks.[28,41] In terms of antimicrobial therapy, symptomatic CAUTIs may be treated with 7 days of appropriate antimicrobials if patients have a prompt resolution of symptoms; therapy should be lengthened to 10 to 14 days for those with a delayed response.[28] Initial empiric therapy should be based on local epidemiologic data regarding causative microorganisms of CAUTIs and antimicrobial resistance patterns. Once culture data become available, antimicrobial therapy should be adjusted as necessary, ideally providing the narrowest spectrum of coverage possible while still providing adequate treatment of the UTI. Symptomatic CAUTIs caused by *Candida* species should be treated with 14 days of antifungal agents.[38]

PREVENTING CAUTIS

General strategies, formulated for the prevention of all HAIs, including strict adherence to hand hygiene, are critical for the prevention of CAUTIs.[42] The urinary tract of hospitalized patients, especially those in an ICU setting, represents a significant reservoir for multidrug-resistant organisms. Therefore, precautions recommended for prevention of transmission of multidrug-resistant organisms should be scrupulously observed in catheterized patients.[43] Limiting unnecessary use of antimicrobials, as part of an overall antimicrobial stewardship program, is another important general strategy to prevent the development of antimicrobial resistance related to urinary catheters.[44]

The measurement and feedback of results of interventions to the clinical care team is an essential component of any improvement program. The CDC NHSN CAUTI rate (symptomatic UTI per 1000 urinary catheter-days) is the most widely accepted measure for CAUTI surveillance and is endorsed by the Infectious Diseases Society of America, the Society of Healthcare Epidemiology of America, and the Association for Professionals in Infection Control and Epidemiology.[28,45,46] In addition, beginning in 2012, the CMS has required as a condition of participation that hospitals, long-term care hospitals, and inpatient rehabilitation facilities submit ICU CAUTI rates to the NHSN. A modified definition of UTI is recommended for surveillance in long-term care facilities.[47] Efforts are currently underway to revise the CDC's NHSN UTI surveillance definitions to improve specificity and clinical relevance of the measure.

However, a population-based measure, using hospital-days as the denominator, has been suggested as an alternative measure to assess improvement interventions at individual hospitals.[48] Other measures, such as rates of asymptomatic bacteriuria, percentage of patients with indwelling catheters, percentage of catheterization with accepted indications, and duration of catheter use, have been used in improvement studies and collaboratives with good success.[49]

Several guidelines with specific recommendations for the prevention of CAUTIs have been developed or recently updated (**Box 1**).[28,45,46,50] However, in 2005, a nationwide survey identified that one-third of hospitals did not conduct surveillance for UTIs, more than one-half did not monitor urinary catheters, and three-quarters did not monitor the duration of catheterization.[12,51] In a follow-up study, after the enactment of the CMS nonpayment rule, still no CAUTI prevention practices had been adopted in more than half of the hospitals, except for the use of bladder

---

Box 1
Strategies for prevention of CAUTIs

Avoid insertion of indwelling urinary catheters

- Placement only for appropriate indications (see **Box 2**)
- Institutional protocols for placement, including perioperative setting

Early removal of indwelling catheters

- Checklist or daily plan
- Nurse-based interventions
- Electronic reminders

Seek alternatives to indwelling catheterization

- Intermittent catheterization
- Condom catheter
- Portable bladder ultrasound scanner

Aseptic techniques for care of catheters

- Sterile insertion
- Closed drainage system
- Maintain gravity drainage
- Avoid routine bladder irrigation

Data from Refs.[28,45,46,50]

ultrasound.[12] Even in ICUs, only a small proportion of surveyed sites had policies supporting bladder ultrasound (26%), catheter removal reminders (12%), or nurse-initiated catheter discontinuation (10%).[52] The systematic adoption of prevention practices has begun to be observed through the use of bundles and collaboratives, as detailed later.[49,53]

A qualitative study of 12 hospitals participating in a statewide program identified barriers to adoption of the key interventions to reduce unnecessary use of urinary catheters. Common barriers included difficulty with nurse and physician engagement, patient and family request for indwelling catheters, and catheter insertion practices and customs in emergency departments.[54] In addition, qualitative studies have revealed that staff variations of the perceived risk and perceived strength of evidence supporting preventive practices should be incorporated into implementation plans.[55,56]

Limiting Use of Urinary Catheters

The foremost strategy for CAUTI prevention is avoidance of or decreasing the duration of urinary catheterization. Catheter utilization varies by ICU type, with the lowest rate in pediatric medical ICUs (0.16 urinary catheter-days/patient-days) and the highest rates reported in trauma ICUs (0.80 urinary catheter-days/patient-days).[16] Decreasing catheter utilization requires interventions at several stages of the lifecycle of the urinary catheter.[26]

The first stage in decreasing catheter utilization is limiting the placement of indwelling urinary catheters. Overall, urinary catheters are overused and the documentation surrounding catheterization is inconsistent[7,57–59]; urinary catheters are placed for inappropriate indications in 21% to 50% of catheterized patients.[7,60] Written policies and criteria for indwelling urinary catheterization, based on accepted indications, is a first step in limiting the placement of urinary catheters; but tracking indications for catheters with feedback to the care team is also important (**Box 2**).[45,50] Some hospitals have had success by targeting interventions for limiting the placement of urinary catheters in emergency departments and operating rooms, locations where the initial placement often takes place.[61]

Box 2
Appropriate indications for indwelling urinary catheters

Acute urinary retention or bladder outlet obstruction

Need for accurate measurements of urinary output

Perioperative use for selected surgical procedures

- Surgical procedures of anticipated long duration

- Urologic procedures

- Intraoperatively for patients with urinary incontinence

- Need for intraoperative urinary monitoring or expected large volume of intravenous infusions

Urinary incontinence in the setting of open perineal or sacral wounds

Improve comfort for end-of-life care or patient preference

Modified from Gould C, Umscheid C, Agarwal R, et al. Healthcare Infection Control Practices Advisory Committee. Guideline for prevention of catheter-associated infections 2009. Infect Control Hosp Epidemiol 2010;31:319–26.

Once catheters are placed, strategies for early removal become necessary to limit the duration of catheterization. Relying on physicians' orders alone may be inadequate for the management of catheters because, in one study, 28% of physicians were unaware that their patient had a catheter.[7] Nurse-driven interventions have demonstrated effectiveness in reducing the duration of catheterization.[62–64] This type of intervention was implemented in a statewide effort that resulted in a significant decrease in catheter use and an increase in appropriate indications of catheters.[49]

Computerized physician order entry systems may offer a more cost-effective and efficient system to reduce both the placement of catheters and the duration of catheterization.[65] A systematic review and meta-analysis found that urinary catheter reminder systems and stop orders seem to reduce the mean duration of catheterization by 37% and CAUTIs by 52%.[66]

Hospitals have also shown success in decreasing urinary catheter prevalence and CAUTIs through the multimodal interventions noted earlier.[67,68] One institution used a multifaceted intervention, which included education, system redesign, rewards, and feedback managed by a dedicated nurse, resulting in a marked decrease in the daily prevalence of urinary catheter days.[67] Strategies to address barriers to the implementation of urinary catheterization bundles include incorporating planned toileting into other patient safety programs, discussing the risk of indwelling urinary catheters with patients and their families, and engaging emergency department personnel to ensure appropriate indications for catheter use are followed have been promoted.[54]

Perioperative Management of Urinary Catheters

Approximately 85% of patients admitted for major surgical procedures have perioperative indwelling catheters. Those patients catheterized longer than 2 days are significantly more likely to develop UTIs and are less likely to be discharged to home.[69] Older surgical patients are at the highest risk for prolonged catheterization; 23% of surgical patients older than 65 years are discharged to skilled nursing facilities with an indwelling catheter in place and have substantially more rehospitalization or deaths within 30 days.[70] Therefore, specific protocols for the management of postoperative urinary catheters are important for reducing urinary catheterization utilization and patient outcomes; the Surgical Care Improvement Project has added the removal of urinary catheters as one of their measures.

In a large prospective trial of patients undergoing orthopedic procedures, patients were entered into the following protocol: (1) limiting catheterization to surgeries of more than 5 hours or for total hip and knee replacements and (2) the removal of urinary catheters on postoperative day 1 after total knee arthroplasty and postoperative day 2 after total hip arthroplasty. This intervention resulted in a two-thirds reduction in the incidence of UTIs.[71]

Alternatives to Indwelling Urinary Catheters

A randomized trial demonstrated a decrease in bacteriuria, symptomatic UTI, or death in patients who used condom catheters when compared with those with indwelling catheters; this benefit was seen primarily in men without dementia.[72] Condom catheters have also been reported to be less painful than indwelling catheters in some men.[72,73] Therefore, condom catheters may be considered in place of indwelling catheters in appropriately selected male patients without urinary retention or bladder outlet obstruction.

Patients with neurogenic bladder and long-term urinary catheters, in particular, may benefit from intermittent catheterization.[50] Intermittent catheterization may also be beneficial for short-term urinary retention. A recent meta-analysis reported a reduced risk of bacteriuria with the use of intermittent catheterization in patients following hip or knee surgery compared with indwelling catheterization.[74] Combining the use of a portable bladder ultrasound scanner with intermittent catheterization may reduce the need for indwelling catheterization.[45,75]

Aseptic Techniques for Insertion and Maintenance of Urinary Catheters

When indwelling catheterization is necessary, aseptic catheter insertion and mainte-nance is recommended for preventing CAUTIs. Urinary catheters should be inserted by a trained health care professional using a sterile technique.[50] Cleaning the meatus before catheter insertion is recommended; but ongoing daily meatal cleaning with an antiseptic has not shown benefit and may increase rates of bacteriuria compared with routine care with soap and water.[50] Sterile lubricant jelly should be used for insertion, but antiseptic lubricants are not necessary.[50]

Maintaining a closed urinary catheter collection system is important to reduce the risk of CAUTIs. Opening the closed system should be avoided, especially when sam-pling urine that may be performed aseptically from a port or from the drainage bag.[50] Prophylactic instillation of antiseptic agents or irrigation of the bladder with antimicro-bial or antiseptic agents has shown no benefit in preventing bacteriuria and is not rec-ommended.[50] Finally, routine exchange of urinary catheters is not recommended except for mechanical reasons because bacteriuria and biofilms return quickly.[2]

Use of Antiinfective Catheters

Antiseptic or antimicrobial impregnated urinary catheters have been studied exten-sively as an adjunctive measure for preventing CAUTIs with variable results.[76,77] How-ever, almost all previous studies used bacteriuria as the primary end point rather than symptomatic UTIs, thus limiting their clinical relevance. In a Cochrane review, silver alloy catheters were found to significantly reduce the incidence of asymptomatic bacteriuria in adult patients catheterized less than 7 days, but the effect was dimin-ished in those catheterized for greater than 7 days.[77] A recent multicenter randomized controlled trial that did use symptomatic CAUTIs as the end point reported no signif-icant clinical benefit with the use of silver alloy-coated or nitrofural-impregnated cath-eters during short-term (<14 days) catheterization.[78] Few studies have evaluated antiseptic and antimicrobial catheters in long-term urinary catheterization.[79] There-fore, there is no recommendation for routine use of antiinfective urinary catheters to prevent CAUTIs.[50] Despite these recommendations, a national study in 2009 revealed that 45% of nonfederal and 22% of Department of Veterans Affairs hospitals used antimicrobial catheters; hospitals using antiinfective catheters often based their deci-sions on hospital-specific pilot studies.[12]

IMPLEMENTATION: THE ROLE OF BUNDLES, COLLABORATIVES, AND LEADERSHIP

Recently, bundles of interventions have been used with success for the prevention of HAIs, including CAUTIs. The Bladder Bundle outlined using the mnemonic *ABCDE* in **Box 3** applied was successfully adopted by the Michigan Hospital Association Keystone initiative.[49,53] After the implementation of this initiative, Michigan hospitals used more key prevention practices and had a lower rate of CAUTIs when compared with hospitals in the rest of the country.[80] Finally, the important role of local hospital leadership and followership for ensuring effective implementation of preventive initia-tives has recently been highlighted.[81–83] The Web site www.catheterout.org provides a list of common barriers along with solutions that hospitals may wish to use in their CAUTI prevention programs.

> **Box 3**
> **The ABCDE for preventing CAUTIs**
>
> - Adherence to general infection control principles (eg, hand hygiene, surveillance and feedback, aseptic insertion, proper maintenance, education) is important.
> - Bladder ultrasound may avoid indwelling catheterization.
> - Condom catheters or other alternatives to an indwelling catheter, such as intermittent catheterization, should be considered in appropriate patients.
> - Do not use the indwelling catheter unless you must.
> - Early removal of the catheter using a reminder or nurse-initiated removal protocol seems to be warranted.
>
> *From* Saint S, Olmsted RN, Fakih MG, et al. Translating health care-associated urinary tract infection prevention research into practice via the bladder bundle. Jt Comm J Qual Patient Saf 2009;35(9):449–55; with permission.

SUMMARY

CAUTIs are common, costly, and cause significant patient morbidity. CAUTIs are associated with hospital pathogens with a high propensity toward antimicrobial resistance. The treatment of asymptomatic CAUTIs accounts for excess antimicrobial use in hospitals and should be avoided. The duration of urinary catheterization is the predominant risk factor for CAUTI; preventive measures directed at limiting the placement and early removal of urinary catheters have a significant impact on decreasing CAUTIs. Bladder bundles, collaboratives, and the support of hospital leaders are powerful tools for implementing appropriate preventive measures against CAUTI.

REFERENCES

1. Chenoweth C, Saint S. Preventing catheter-associated urinary tract infections in the intensive care unit. Crit Care Clin 2013;29:19–32.
2. Chenoweth CE, Saint S. Urinary tract infections. Infect Dis Clin North Am 2011; 25(1):103–15.
3. Nicolle L. Urinary catheter-associated infections. Infect Dis Clin North Am 2012; 26:13–27.
4. Burton D, Edwards J, Srinivasan A, et al. Trends in catheter-associated urinary tract infection in adult intensive care units-United States, 1990–2007. Infect Control Hosp Epidemiol 2011;32:748–56.
5. Weber D, Sickbert-Bennett E, Gould C, et al. Incidence of catheter-associated and non-catheter-associated urinary tract infections in a healthcare system. Infect Control Hosp Epidemiol 2011;32(8):822–3.
6. Saint S, Lipsky BA. Preventing catheter-related bacteriuria: should we? Can we? How? Arch Intern Med 1999;159(8):800–8.
7. Saint S, Wiese J, Amory JK, et al. Are physicians aware of which of their patients have indwelling catheters? Am J Med 2000;109:476–80.
8. Sorbye L, Finne-Soveri H, Ljunggren G, et al. Indwelling catheter use in home care: elderly, aged 65+, in 11 countries in Europe. Age Ageing 2005;34(4): 377–81.
9. Chang R, Green MT, Chenoweth CE, et al. Epidemiology of hospital-acquired urinary tract-related bloodstream infection at a university hospital. Infect Control Hosp Epidemiol 2011;32(11):1127–9.

10. Shuman EK, Chenoweth CE. Recognition and prevention of healthcare-associated urinary tract infections in the intensive care unit. Crit Care Med 2010;38:S373–9.
11. Saint S, Meddings JA, Calfee D, et al. Catheter-associated urinary tract infection and the Medicare rule changes. Ann Intern Med 2009;150(12):877–84.
12. Krein S, Kowalski C, Hofer TP, et al. Preventing hospital-acquired infections: a national survey of practices reported by U.S. hospitals in 2005 and 2009. J Gen Intern Med 2012;27:773–9.
13. Lee G, Kleinman K, Soumerai S, et al. Effect of nonpayment for preventable infections in U.S. hospitals. N Engl J Med 2012;36:1428–37.
14. Meddings JA, Reichert H, Rogers MA, et al. Effect of nonpayment for hospital-acquired, catheter-associate urinary tract infection: a statewide analysis. Ann Intern Med 2012;157(5):305–12.
15. Umsheid C, Mitchell M, Doshi J, et al. Estimating the proportion of healthcare-associated infections that are reasonably preventable and the related mortality and costs. Infect Control Hosp Epidemiol 2011;32(2):101–14.
16. Dudeck M, Horan T, Peterson K, et al. National Healthcare Safety Network (NHSN) report, data summary for 2010, device-associated module. Am J Infect Control 2011;39:798–816.
17. Langley JM, Hanakowski M, LeBlanc JC. Unique epidemiology of nosocomial urinary tract infection in children. Am J Infect Control 2001;29:94–8.
18. Tambyah PA, Halvorson KT, Maki DG. A prospective study of pathogenesis of catheter-associated urinary tract infections. Mayo Clin Proc 1999;74:131–6.
19. Saint S, Chenoweth CE. Biofilms and catheter-associated urinary tract infections. Infect Dis Clin North Am 2003;17:411–32.
20. Chitnis A, Edwards J, Ricks P, et al. Device-associated infection rates, device utilization, and antimicrobial resistance in long-term acute care hospitals reporting to the National Healthcare Safety Network, 2010. Infect Control Hosp Epidemiol 2012;33(10):993–1000.
21. Sievert D, Ricks P, Edwards J, et al. Antimicrobial-resistant pathogens associated with healthcare-associated infections: summary of data reported to the National Healthcare Safety Network at the Centers for Disease Control and Prevention, 2009-2010. Infect Control Hosp Epidemiol 2013;34(1):1–14.
22. Bouza E, San Juan R, Munoz P, et al. European perspective on nosocomial urinary tract infections. I. Report on the microbiology workload, etiology and antimicrobial susceptibility (ESGNI-003 study). Clin Microbiol Infect 2001;7:523–31.
23. Sobel JD, Kauffman CA, McKinsey D, et al. Candiduria: a randomized, double-blind study of treatment with fluconazole and placebo. Clin Infect Dis 2000;30:19–24.
24. Demuth PJ, Gerding DN, Crossley K. Staphylococcus aureus bacteriuria. Arch Intern Med 1979;139:78–80.
25. Donlan RM. Biofilms and device-associated infections. Emerg Infect Dis 2001;7(2):1–4.
26. Meddings J, Saint S. Disrupting the life cycle of the urinary catheter. Clin Infect Dis 2011;52:1291–3.
27. Greene MT, Chang R, Kuhn L, et al. Predictors of hospital-acquired urinary tract-related bloodstream infection. Infect Control Hosp Epidemiol 2012;33(10):1001–7.
28. Hooten T, Bradley S, Cardenas D, et al. Diagnosis, prevention and treatment of catheter-associated urinary tract infection in adults: 2009 international clinical

practice guidelines from the Infectious Diseases Society of America. Clin Infect Dis 2010;50:625–63.

29. Musher DM, Thorsteinsson SB, Airola VM II. Quantitative urinalysis: diagnosing urinary tract infection in men. JAMA 1976;236:2069–72.

30. Tambyah PA, Maki DG. Catheter-associated urinary tract infection is rarely symptomatic: a prospective study of 1,497 catheterized patients. Arch Intern Med 2000;160(5):678–82.

31. Tambyah PA, Maki DG. The relationship between pyuria and infection in patients with indwelling urinary catheters: a prospective study of 761 patients. Arch Intern Med 2000;160(5):673–7.

32. Stark RP, Maki DG. Bacteriuria in the catheterized patient. What quantitative level of bacteriuria is relevant? N Engl J Med 1984;311(9):560–4.

33. Anonymous. The prevention and management of urinary tract infections among people with spinal cord injuries. National Institute on Disabilities and Rehabilitation Research Consensus Statement. January 27-29, 1992. J Am Paraplegia Soc 1992;15(3):194–204.

34. Cope M, Cevallos M, Cadle R, et al. Inappropriate treatment of catheter-associated asymptomatic bacteriuria in a tertiary care hospital. Clin Infect Dis 2009;48(9):1182–8.

35. Gandhi T, Flanders S, Markovitz E, et al. Importance of urinary tract infection to antibiotic use among hospitalized patients. Infect Control Hosp Epidemiol 2009; 30:193–5.

36. Trautner B, Kelly P, Petersen N, et al. A hospital-site controlled intervention using audit and feedback to implement guidelines concerning inappropriate treatment of catheter-associated asymptomatic bacteriuria. Implement Sci 2011;6:41.

37. Nicolle L, Bradley S, Colgan R, et al. Infectious Diseases Society of America guidelines for the diagnosis and treatment of asymptomatic bacteriuria in adults. Clin Infect Dis 2005;40:643–54.

38. Pappas P, Kauffman C, Andes D, et al. Clinical practice guidelines for the management of candidiasis: 2009 update by the Infectious Diseases Society of America. Clin Infect Dis 2009;48:503–35.

39. Harding G, Nicolle L, Ronald A, et al. How long should catheter-acquired urinary tract infection in women be treated? A randomized controlled study. Ann Intern Med 1991;114(9):713–9.

40. Pavese P, Saurel N, Labarere J, et al. Does an educational session with an infectious diseases physician reduce the use of inappropriate antibiotic therapy for inpatients with positive urine culture results? A controlled before-and-after study. Infect Control Hosp Epidemiol 2009;30(6):596–9.

41. Raz R, Schiller D, Nicolle LE. Chronic indwelling catheter replacement before antimicrobial therapy for symptomatic urinary tract infection. J Urol 2000; 164(4):1254–8.

42. Boyce J, Pittet D. Guideline for hand hygiene in health-care settings. Recommendations of the Healthcare Infection Control Practices Advisory Committee and the HICPAC/SHEA/APIC/IDSA Hand Hygiene Task Force. MMWR Recomm Rep 2002;51(RR-16):1–45.

43. Siegel JD, Rhinehart E, Jackson M, et al, Healthcare Infection Control Practices Advisory Committee. Management of multidrug-resistant organisms in health care settings, 2006. Am J Infect Control 2007;35(10 Suppl 2):S165–93.

44. Dellit T, Owens R, McGowan J Jr, et al. Infectious Diseases Society of America and the Society for Healthcare Epidemiology of America guidelines for

developing an institutional program to enhance antimicrobial stewardship. Clin Infect Dis 2007;44:159–77.

45. Lo E, Nicolle L, Classen D, et al. Strategies to prevent catheter-associated urinary tract infections in acute care hospitals. Infect Control Hosp Epidemiol 2008;29:S41–50.

46. Rebmann T, Greene L. Preventing catheter-associated urinary tract infections: an executive summary of the Association for Professionals in Infection Control and Epidemiology. Am J Infect Control 2010;38:644–6.

47. Stone N, Ashraf M, Calder J, et al. Surveillance definitions of infections in long-term care facilities: revisiting the McGeer criteria. Infect Control Hosp Epidemiol 2012;33(10):965–77.

48. Fakih M, Greene T, Kennedy E, et al. Introducing a population-based outcome measure to evaluate the effect of interventions to reduce catheter-associated infection. Am J Infect Control 2012;40:359–64.

49. Fakih MG, Watson SR, Greene MT, et al. Reducing inappropriate urinary catheter use: a statewide effort. Arch Intern Med 2012;172(3):255–60.

50. Gould C, Umscheid C, Agarwal R, et al, Healthcare Infection Control Practices Advisory Committee. Guideline for prevention of catheter-associated infections 2009. Infect Control Hosp Epidemiol 2010;31:319–26.

51. Saint S, Kowalski CP, Kaufman SR, et al. Preventing hospital-acquired urinary tract infection in the United States: a national study. Clin Infect Dis 2008;46(2):243–50.

52. Conway L, Pogorzelska M, Larson E, et al. Adoption of policies to prevent catheter-associated urinary tract infections in United States intensive care units. Am J Infect Control 2012;40(8):705–10.

53. Saint S, Olmsted RN, Fakih MG, et al. Translating health care-associated urinary tract infection prevention research into practice via the bladder bundle. Jt Comm J Qual Patient Saf 2009;35(9):449–55.

54. Krein S, Kowalski C, Harrod M, et al. Barriers to reducing urinary catheter use: a qualitative assessment of a statewide initiative. JAMA Intern Med 2013;173(10):881–6.

55. Harrod M, Kowalski C, Saint S, et al. Variation in risk perceptions: a qualitative study of why unnecessary urinary catheter use continues to be problematic. BMC Health Serv Res 2013;13:151.

56. Saint S, Greene M, Olmsted R, et al. Perceived strength of evidence supporting practices to prevent health care-associated infection: results from a national survey of infection prevention personnel. Am J Infect Control 2013;41:100–6.

57. Conybeare A, Pathak S, Imam I. The quality of hospital records of urethral catheterisation. Ann R Coll Surg Engl 2002;84(2):109–10.

58. Gardam MA, Amihod B, Orenstein P, et al. Overutilization of indwelling urinary catheters and the development of nosocomial urinary tract infections. Clin Perform Qual Health Care 1998;6:99–102.

59. Jain P, Parada JP, David A, et al. Overuse of the indwelling urinary tract catheter in hospitalized medical patients. Arch Intern Med 1995;155(13):1425–9.

60. Munasinghe RL, Yazdani H, Siddique M, et al. Appropriateness of use of indwelling urinary catheters in patients admitted to the medical service. Infect Control Hosp Epidemiol 2001;22(10):647–9.

61. Fakih MG, Pena M, Shemes S, et al. Effect of establishing guidelines on appropriate urinary catheter placement. Acad Emerg Med 2010;17(3):337–40.

62. Fakih MG, Dueweke C, Meisner S, et al. Effect of nurse-led multidisciplinary rounds on reducing the unnecessary use of urinary catheterization in hospitalized patients. Infect Control Hosp Epidemiol 2008;29(8):815–9.

63. Huang WC, Wann SR, Lin SL, et al. Catheter-associated urinary tract infections in intensive care units can be reduced by prompting physicians to remove unnecessary catheters. Infect Control Hosp Epidemiol 2004;25(11):974–8.

64. Saint S, Kaufman SR, Thompson M, et al. A reminder reduces urinary catheterization in hospitalized patients. Jt Comm J Qual Patient Saf 2005;31(8):455–62.

65. Cornia PB, Amory JK, Fraser S, et al. Computer-based order entry decreases duration of indwelling urinary catheterization in hospitalized patients. Am J Med 2003;114:404–6.

66. Meddings J, Rogers MA, Macy M, et al. Systematic review and meta-analysis: reminder systems to reduce catheter-associated urinary tract infections and urinary catheter use in hospitalized patients. Clin Infect Dis 2010;2010:550–60.

67. Knoll B, Wright D, Ellingson L, et al. Reduction of inappropriate urinary catheter use at a Veterans Affairs hospital through a multifaceted quality improvement project. Clin Infect Dis 2011;52(11):1283–90.

68. Miller B, Krein S, Fowler K, et al. A multimodal intervention to reduce urinary catheter use and associated infection at a Veterans Affairs Medical Center. Infect Control Hosp Epidemiol 2013;34(6):631–3.

69. Wald HL, Ma A, Bratzler DW, et al. Indwelling urinary catheter use in the postoperative period: analysis of the national surgical infection prevention project data. Arch Surg 2008;143(6):551–7.

70. Wald HL, Epstein AM, Radcliff TA, et al. Extended use of urinary catheters in older surgical patients: a patient safety problem? Infect Control Hosp Epidemiol 2008;29(2):116–24.

71. Stephan F, Sax H, Wachsmuth M, et al. Reduction of urinary tract infection and antibiotic use after surgery: a controlled, prospective, before-after intervention study. Clin Infect Dis 2006;42(11):1544–51.

72. Saint S, Kaufman SR, Rogers MA, et al. Condom versus indwelling urinary catheters: a randomized trial. J Am Geriatr Soc 2006;54(7):1055–61.

73. Saint S, Lipsky BA, Baker PD, et al. Urinary catheters: what type do men and their nurses prefer? J Am Geriatr Soc 1999;47(12):1453–7.

74. Niël-Weise B, van den Broek PJ. Urinary catheter policies for short-term bladder drainage in adults. Cochrane Database of Systematic Reviews 2005;(3):CD004203. http://dx.doi.org/10.1002/14651858.CD004203.pub2.

75. Stevens E. Bladder ultrasound: avoiding unnecessary catheterizations. Medsurg Nurs 2005;14(4):249–53.

76. Johnson JR, Kuskowski MA, Wilt TJ. Systematic review: antimicrobial urinary catheters to prevent catheter-associated urinary tract infection in hospitalized patients. Ann Intern Med 2006;144(2):116–26.

77. Schumm K, Lam T. Types of urethral catheters for management of short-term voiding problems in hospitalised adults. Cochrane Database Syst Rev 2008;(2):CD004013.

78. Pickard R, Lam T, MacLennan G, et al. Antimicrobial catheters for reduction of symptomatic urinary tract infection in adults requiring short-term catheterisation in hospital: a multicentre randomised controlled trial. Lancet 2012;380:1927–35.

79. Jahn P, Preuss M, Kernig A, et al. Types of indwelling urinary catheters for long-term bladder drainage in adults. Cochrane Database Syst Rev 2007;(3):CD004997.

80. Saint S, Greene M, Kowalski C, et al. Preventing catheter-associated urinary tract infection in the United States; a national comparative study. JAMA Intern Med 2013;173(10):874–9.
81. Damschroder L, Banaszak-Holl J, Kowalski CP, et al. The role of the champion in infection prevention: results from a multistate qualitative study. Qual Saf Health Care 2009;18:434–40.
82. Saint S, Kowalski CP, Banaszak-Holl J, et al. How active resisters and organizational constipators affect health care-acquired infection prevention efforts. Jt Comm J Qual Patient Saf 2009;35(5):239–46.
83. Saint S, Kowalski CP, Banaszak-Holl J, et al. The importance of leadership in preventing healthcare-associated infection: results of a multisite qualitative study. Infect Control Hosp Epidemiol 2010;31(9):901–7.

Management of Non-catheter-associated Complicated Urinary Tract Infection

Elodi J. Dielubanza, MD*, Daniel J. Mazur, MD,
Anthony J. Schaeffer, MD

KEYWORDS

- Urinary tract infection • UTI • Complicated UTI • Upper tract infection
- UTI in pregnancy • Renal abscess • Perirenal abscess • Prostatitis

KEY POINTS

- A urinary tract infection (UTI) is considered complicated when it occurs in the setting of a structural or functional abnormality of the urinary tract, a compromised host (eg, diabetes, immunosuppression), pregnancy, or as a result of bacteria with increased virulence and antimicrobial resistance. UTI in men and boys should be considered complicated until proven otherwise.
- Initial evaluation of a patient with a suspected complicated UTI includes a detailed history, physical examination, urinalysis, and urine culture, as well as imaging.
- The selection of imaging modality should depend on the clinical condition of the patient, the clinical question to be answered by the study, and the strengths and limitations of the modality.
- In the setting of UTI with genitourinary tract obstruction, prompt urologic consultation is warranted for prompt decompression.
- UTI in pregnancy should be taken seriously given the risk of pyelonephritis and its associated morbidity for mother and fetus. Pregnant women should be screened and treated for asymptomatic bacteriuria to decrease this risk.

INTRODUCTION

Urinary tract infection (UTI) is an inflammatory response to the invasion of the urothelium by a pathogenic organism, resulting in a wide range of upper and lower urinary tract disease. It is one of the most commonly encountered infectious diseases worldwide, and as such, one of the most common reasons for outpatient medical

---

Funding Sources: Dr A.J. Schaeffer: Nil.
Conflicts of Interest: Dr A.J. Schaeffer: Nil.
Department of Urology, Feinberg School of Medicine, Northwestern University, 303 East Chicago Avenue, Chicago, IL 60611, USA
* Corresponding author.
E-mail address: e-dielubanza@northwestern.edu

Infect Dis Clin N Am 28 (2014) 121–134
http://dx.doi.org/10.1016/j.idc.2013.10.005
0891-5520/14/$ – see front matter © 2014 Elsevier Inc. All rights reserved.

id.theclinics.com

evaluation. In the United States alone, UTI is the chief complaint in 8 million clinic and emergency department visits.[1] Most UTIs are uncomplicated, self-limited infections, which are confined to the bladder and effectively treated with short-course, empiric antimicrobials. Conversely, complicated infections occur in the setting of structural or functional abnormalities, a compromised host (ie, pregnant, diabetic), or causative bacteria with increased virulence or antimicrobial resistance. UTI in men and boys should be considered complicated until proper evaluation proves otherwise. There is a significant increase in the morbidity and mortality associated with complicated infections, ranging from loss of renal function to sepsis and death, so timely recognition is vitally important. Structural and functional abnormalities may be known before infection, but often, patients present with an infection whose clinical features are merely suggestive of unrecognized abnormalities. Therefore, care of these patients can be a significant clinical challenge. Provided, is a guide to enable the treating physician to maintain an appropriate index of suspicion, select the optimal diagnostic and imaging tests that would lead to quick and accurate diagnosis of complicated UTI, and institute effective therapy, to minimize morbidity.

DIAGNOSING A COMPLICATED UTI
Understanding the Natural Defense of the Genitourinary System

The natural antegrade flow of urine through the genitourinary system is its greatest defense against pathogenic intruders. Virtually all complicated infections result from an impairment in the ability to "flush" out microorganisms. All conditions that promote complicated UTI do so by disrupting antegrade urine flow, causing structural or functional obstruction, or contributing to nidus formation. Obstruction to urinary drainage can lead to changes in intrarenal blood flow, decreasing delivery of agents of the body's humoral defenses as well as antimicrobials. Retrograde flow of urine, both by physiologic reflux and by instrumentation, allow for inoculation of the upper urinary tract. The presence of any static agent in the urinary tract, be it urine, foreign body, or stone, provides residence for pathogens as well as fortress against effective antimicrobial therapy. Understanding this concept is an excellent starting point to inform which clinical questions you will ask in an evaluation and how you may choose to go about answering them.

History and Physical Examination

Initial evaluation with history and physical examination is a primary tool in the timely recognition of complicated UTI. It should elucidate pre-existing or potential complicating factors, exclude other causes of genitourinary symptoms, and identify patients at risk for significant morbidity associated with infection (**Box 1**). The most common symptoms of uncomplicated UTI are dysuria, urgency, and frequency. Suprapubic pain and hematuria can be present as well, although less often. Clinical signs and symptoms that should heighten concern for complicated infection include flank pain, fever, and other signs systemic inflammatory response syndrome, like hypotension. A thorough medical history should include assessment of pregnancy status, structural and functional genitourinary abnormalities, kidney stones, renal insufficiency, immune deficiency, pelvic surgery, diabetes mellitus, neurologic disorders, as well as any recent antibiotic use, hospitalization, or genitourinary instrumentation. A pertinent physical examination must include vital signs, an abdominal and flank examination to assess for tenderness, a full external genital examination in men and women, and a limited pelvic examination in women to assess for evidence of pelvic organ prolapse or urethral diverticula.

| **Box1** |
| **Does a patient have a complicated UTI?** |

Has a complicated UTI

- Structural or functional abnormality of urinary tract
- Genitourinary obstruction (eg, stone)
- Pregnancy
- Immunosuppression
- Diabetes
- Renal insufficiency
- Indwelling or intermittent catheter use
- Fever (eg, possible pyelonephritis or renal abscess)

Likely has a complicated UTI (until ruled out)

- Men
- Children or history of childhood UTI
- Nosocomial or nursing home–acquired infection
- Recent antimicrobial use
- Recent urinary tract instrumentation
- Prolonged symptoms (>7 days)

Conversion from uncomplicated to complicated UTI

- Symptoms fail to respond to appropriate therapy
- Failure to eradicate bacteria after appropriate therapy

Laboratory Evaluation

Urinalysis with microscopic evaluation (UA), urine culture and sensitivity, and serum chemistry should be performed in all patients in whom you suspect complicated UTI. Urine specimens should be obtained via careful clean-catch, mid -stream technique. If UA is suggestive of contamination (ie, presence of epithelial cells on microscopy) or the patient is unable to void, a catheterized specimen should be obtained. Urine culture is essential in pathogen identification, antibiotic selection, and confirmation of cure and thus should be performed before, during, and after therapy. Serum chemistry will reveal electrolyte anomalies that may be suggestive of an obstructive process, evidence of poorly controlled diabetes, and impaired renal function that may decrease the efficacy of antimicrobial therapy. Complete blood count should be performed in patients present with fever to assess for leukocytosis. Blood culture may be reserved for the clinically unstable with fever and hypotension.

Imaging

Radiographic imaging is an essential component of the workup. It is performed to identify evidence of hydronephrosis, urinary stones, and aberrant anatomy. A variety of imaging studies can provide delineation of anatomic features that make an individual susceptible to infection and render therapeutic overtures ineffective. However, selection of the most appropriate imaging modality can be daunting. In making this decision, first, consider the acuity of the patient's clinical status and next remember that the chosen modality should be sufficient to fully evaluate the conditions for which one has clinical suspicion. Knowing the strengths and limitations of each modality is extremely helpful in that regard. Renal and bladder ultrasound, noncontrast computed tomography (CT), and contrast-enhanced CT are each excellent for evaluating the genitourinary tract, although each has diagnostic limitations and tradeoffs.

Ultrasound allows for evaluation of the renal parenchyma for evidence of atrophy, solid or cystic lesions, or collecting system duplication. It can reveal renal and bladder calculi, collecting system dilation (ie, hydronephrosis) abnormalities of the bladder wall (ie, diverticula), and elevated postvoid residual urine volume. The main limitation of this modality is its difficulty in identifying ureteral stones, especially in distal locations. Otherwise, ultrasound is inexpensive and widely available and spares the patient ionizing radiation exposure. Furthermore, it should be considered the first-line modality in the evaluation of pregnant patients. Any findings suggestive of parenchymal mass or noncalculus collecting system filling defect should prompt follow-up imaging with contrast CT, magnetic resonance imaging, and/or cystoscopy and ureteroscopy as indicated.

Noncontrast CT also offers good anatomic detail of the renal parenchyma and collecting system and well as other intra-abdominal structures, allowing for the evaluation for alternative diagnoses of abdominal or flank pain. It can localize even minute renal or ureteral stones and is considered the gold standard for evaluation for nephrolithiasis. Its main diagnostic limitation is in poor characterization of solid or heterogeneous renal lesions and noncalculous collecting system filling defects. If such a lesion is identified, a contrast-enhanced CT or magnetic resonance imaging is warranted.

Contrast-enhanced CT offers superior anatomic detail for evaluation of the kidneys and all other intra-abdominal organs, and good characterization of solid and complex renal lesions. In addition, the extent of contrast uptake by the renal parenchyma can provide a gross assessment of function in each renal unit. The diagnostic limitation of this study is that urinary calculi can be obscured if contrast is within the collecting system at the time that images are acquired. Patients must have normal creatinine and no pertinent allergies to receive iodinated contrast. All CT studies involve exposure to ionizing radiation.

Ultimately, selection of the optimal imaging modality requires a balance between limitations and risks of each modality with the clinical benefit derived from the timeliest diagnosis.

Empiric Therapy and Next Steps

Prompt initiation of empiric, broad-spectrum antibiosis is vitally important in the initial approach to patients with complicated UTI. It can help to contain the invading pathogen and reduce the risk of systemic infection and the associated morbidity. Selected agents should offer good coverage of the most common uropathogens, *Eschericha coli*, and enterobacteriaceae species. Fluoroquinolones and third-generation cephalosporins are good choices. Oral therapy is appropriate for clinically stable patients who are able to tolerate medications by mouth. Clinically ill patients and those unable to tolerate oral intake should be started on intravenous antimicrobials. Whether the clinical scenario warrants inpatient or outpatient management, careful monitoring is mandatory. Clinical status can change rapidly, so the patient should maintain close contact with the physician until confirmation that the infection has resolved.

Positive findings on the initial evaluation or failure to respond to appropriate therapy after a normal evaluation are indications urologic consultation (**Fig. 1**).

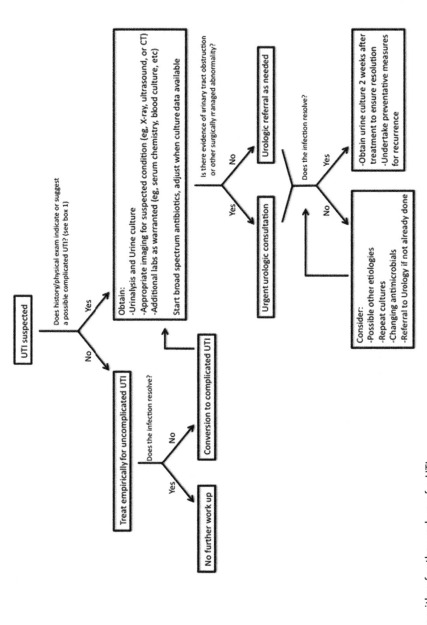

Fig. 1. Algorithm for the workup of a UTI.

APPROACH TO SPECIFIC COMPLICATED INFECTIONS
Acute Pyelonephritis

Pyelonephritis is an ascending UTI that has reached the level of the renal pelvis. Upper tract infection in itself does not necessarily constitute a complicated UTI; uncomplicated pyelonephritis can occur in healthy, anatomically normal patients. However, each case should be considered complicated until proven otherwise. Clinically, it is characterized by fever, flank pain with costovertebral angle tenderness, positive UA, and elevated serum white blood cell count. The development of pyelonephritis usually depends on bacterial capacity for ascent as well compromise in host anatomic defenses to facilitate colonization and traverse of the lengthy ureter without washout. Clustering of disease in states, which permit retrograde flow of urine or impair renal drainage, like pregnancy and vesicourteral reflux, supports this assertion. However, cystitis-associated inflammatory changes in the bladder may be sufficient to induce a transient reflux and enhance the potential for upper tract involvement, so affected persons may not have durable anatomic abnormalities.[2] It is essential that individuals presenting with pyelonephritis receive imaging that identifies or excludes anatomic factors that could lead to recurrent episodes, as this will affect the mode of therapy. In the presence of obstruction, significant medical comorbidities, or systemic signs of illness, hospital admission with hemodynamic monitoring, and intravenous hydration and antibiotics are indicated.

In healthy patients who are clinically well without overt signs of obstruction, a 7-day course of empiric oral fluoroquinolones is a reasonable approach.[3] Any patient who is managed on an outpatient basis should be reliable for follow-up in case alterations to antimicrobial regimen are necessary after final culture results, or fever fails to respond after 72 hours. In addition, every patient should receive a follow-up urine culture after completion of the antimicrobial regimen, to ensure eradication.

Pregnancy

Pregnancy is an independent risk factor of upper UTI. The morbidity associated with these infections is significant; large retrospective studies have shown an increased rate of prematurity, low birth weight, preeclampsia, and cesarean delivery in affected women.[4] As such, screening and treatment of asymptomatic bacteriuria is the standard of care in this population. Although the incidence of asymptomatic bacteriuria remains virtually identical in pregnant and nonpregnant women of childbearing age (2%–7%), pregnancy-induced physiologic changes in the urinary tract increase the likelihood of symptomatic infection. Progesterone induces tonic relaxation of the ureteric smooth muscle, while blood volume and glomerular filtration rate are markedly increased, creating a permissive environment for renal pelviceal and ureteral dilation, vesicoureteral reflux, and urinary stasis. Therefore, 25% to 40% of pregnant women with untreated bacteriuria will develop pyelonephritis. Previous history of UTI, low socioeconomic status, indigence, intercurrent diabetes, and sickle cell trait further increase this risk. Sterilizing the urine with short-course antimicrobials can reduce the incidence of pyelonephritis by 75%.[5–8] A 3-day course of culture directed therapy with a β-lactam or nitrofurantoin is effective for both asymptomatic bacteriuria and symptomatic lower urinary infections. A follow-up culture after the completion of therapy is imperative to confirm pathogen eradication.

Patients with clinical signs consistent with pyelonephritis should be admitted for parenteral antimicrobials and hemodynamic and obstetric monitoring (if gestational age warrants), because preterm labor can be induced by systemic infection. Antimicrobial therapy should include a third-generation cephalosporin, gentamicin, or aztreonam. Patients should receive imaging with ultrasound to exclude obstruction. Patients without obstruction, who respond to therapy and remain stable, can be discharged with a 14- to 21-day course of culture-directed therapy. Patients with evidence of concurrent obstruction and/or those who fail to respond may require additional imaging or intervention. Low-dose noncontrast CT can be used if a nonvisualized urinary calculus is suspected, although the patient should be thoroughly counseled on the risk of ionizing radiation exposure in pregnancy. Decompression with ureteral stent or percutaneous nephrostomy tube (PCN) should be undertaken if imaging confirms obstructing calculus. Drainage should be maintained until after delivery or until definitive therapy can be completed. The patient should remain on antimicrobial therapy for as long as stents or PCN remain in place, as bacterial colonization is common. Most practitioners opt for management of obstruction with stents or PCN in the pregnant population; however, rapid encrustation necessitates exchange every 6 weeks and irritative voiding symptoms are not uncommon. More frequently, urologists are reporting good outcomes with the treatment of obstructing stones in pregnant women with ureteroscopy with either ultrasound or limited fluoroscopy.[9]

Nephrolithiasis

Nephrolithiasis is one of the most common urologic conditions with a prevalence of 10% to 15% within the United States.[10,11] UTI can be both a causative and a complicating factor in urinary stone disease, although the latter is certainly more common. Most calculi are thought to form secondary to dehydration and low urine volumes, although 10% to 15% of stones form because of infection with stone-promoting pathogens.[12] Urease-producing bacteria, such as *Proteus* and *Klebisella*, split urea into ammonia and carbon dioxide, leading to subsequent conversion to ammonium and bicarbonate, respectively, and alkalinization of the urine. Elevated urine pH promotes the precipitation magnesium ammonium phosphate as well as mucoproteins and mucopolysaccharides, giving rise to Struvite and Matrix stones, respectively. These "infection stones" may be suspected in a patient with alkaline urine, chronic flank pain, and recurrent UTI at short intervals, particularly the same with urease-producing organisms.

UTI can complicate existing stone disease when a calculus becomes secondarily colonized and acts as a nidus for uropathogens and/or causes obstruction of the urinary tract. Colonized stones most often translate clinically into recurrent UTI or pyelonephritis. If an element of obstruction develops in this setting, the clinical scenario can become grave, characterized by sepsis or even abscess formation. Symptoms are variable; patients may present with dysuria, urgency and frequency, hematuria, localizing flank pain, nausea and vomiting, fever, or hemodynamic instability. In any patient in whom UTI complicated by urolithiasis is suspected, it is important to ascertain personal or family history of stones, recurrent UTI, and metabolic disorders or malabsorptive disorders. UA often reveals the nonspecific pyuria, bacteriuria, hematuria, but may provide a helpful clue if the urine pH is less than 6.0 or greater than 7.5. Urine culture may reveal stone-promoting pathogens. Leukocytosis, creatinine elevation, and fever should certainly raise suspicion for an upper tract infection. Imaging is the only method to confirm this diagnosis and noncontrast CT scan is the gold standard. It offers the most accurate localization of stone, allows for assessment of the renal parenchyma, reveals evidence of obstruction, and can offer an opportunity to evaluate for alternative diagnosis. If CT is unavailable, renal and bladder ultrasound with kidney/ureters/bladder radiograph may be used. However, ultrasound may not demonstrate small, nonshadowing stones or ureteral stones and kidney/ureters/bladder radiograph will not demonstrate small or radiolucent stones.

If an obstructive stone is identified in the presence of UTI, immediate urologic consultation is warranted for decompression of the collecting system with indwelling ureteral stent or PCN. In setting of nonobstructive stones and evidence of UTI, empiric antibiotic therapy is required. The choice of oral versus parenteral therapy is based on the clinical scenario. If the patient is clinically well, outpatient antibiotic therapy is acceptable, although urologic consultation for management of stones should be initiated.

Ultimately, definitive therapy for stones is indicated to ensure resolution of obstruction and to eradicate the nidus for recurrent infection. However, intervention should be deferred until the urinary tract can be adequately sterilized with antimicrobials, which may require the patient to remain on therapy until the necessary procedures can be completed to limit the risk of systemic seeding of urinary pathogens during urologic procedures in which positive pressure irrigation is used in the upper urinary tract.

Renal and Perirenal Abscess

Abscess formation is an infrequent manifestation of upper UTI, with a reported incidence of 1 in 10,000 in the literature.[13,14] A renal abscess is a collection of purulent fluid within the renal parenchyma, confined by the renal capsule. Perirenal abscess is a collection of purulent fluid outside of the renal capsule but is confined by Gerota fascia, often resulting from rupture of acute cortical abscess or renal pelvis during containing an evolving suppurative infection, superinfection of perinephric hematoma, or by hematogenous spread from an extrarenal site. The functionally and anatomically normal kidney is adept at combating suppurative infection; therefore, abscesses are most often noted in the setting of recent genitourinary instrumentation, tubular obstruction, renal calculi, or parenchymal injury. Today, the most common causative organisms are ascending gram-negative bacteria from the lower urinary tract. Before the modern antimicrobial era and widespread use of antibiotics, the most common cause was gram-positive bacteria via hematogenous spread from a nonurinary source, usually skin. Currently, abscess formation from hematogenous seeding occurs rarely but is most often perirenal in location and associated with intravenous drug use or antecedent extrarenal infection with multi-drug-resistant bacteria. Compromised immune status also plays a role in risk for abscess formation. In the literature, 30% to 50% of these infections occur in persons with diabetes mellitus.[13–15]

Maintaining a high level of clinical suspicion for renal or perirenal abscess in patients with risk factors is crucial, because the mortality from unrecognized abscess has been as high as 50%.

The clinical presentation can be diverse, although often includes fever, malaise, flank and/or abdominal pain, with or without symptoms of cystitis. Patients may have presented earlier with a seemingly uncomplicated pyelonephritis that has failed to respond to appropriate therapy. Laboratory evaluations are likely to show leukocytosis, whereas UA and urine culture may be negative unless the abscess cavity is in contact with the urinary collecting system. Blood cultures are most often positive only if the causative organism is a gram-positive bacterium. Clinical suspicion for abscess should be high in any patient with persistent fever, localizing pain, and leukocytosis, especially if these findings persist despite a trial of antibiotics.

Imaging is the mainstay of diagnosis, and ultrasound and CT are acceptable modalities, although CT is the gold standard. Ultrasound will reveal a hypoechoic mass that may contain septa. CT offers superior anatomic detail as well as the opportunity to identify extrarenal infectious process and reveals well-circumscribed mass with low-attenuating core and an enhancing rim.

Intravenous antibiosis is the centerpiece of therapy for these lesions, and drainage may be indicated depending on the size and characteristics of the abscess, the clinical scenario, and the patient's comorbidities. For lesions less than 3 cm, an initial trial of intravenous antibiotics with close monitoring for clinical improvement can be tried if the patient is clinically stable, without immunocompromising conditions. For lesions that measure 3 to 5 cm or contain gas, patients with immunodeficiency, or clinical instability, percutaneous drainage should be strongly considered at presentation. Percutaneous drainage has been shown to be effective in the literature with a small minority necessitating additional procedures for drainage. Historically, surgical drainage was advocated for lesions greater than 5 cm; however, many surgeons are opting for an initial trial percutaneous drainage, with operative intervention only in the setting of failure percutaneous drainage. Nephrectomy should be considered in the setting of a nonfunctioning affected kidney.[5,13]

Neurogenic Bladder

Neurogenic bladder is a dysfunction of the bladder secondary to disease of the central nervous system or peripheral nerves involved in the control of micturition. Clinically, it can give rise to inefficient voiding contractions with incomplete bladder emptying, elevated residual urine volume, and increased bladder storage pressures with resultant vesicoureteral reflux and hydronephrosis. Neurogenic changes to the bladder can complicate several clinical conditions in addition to the classically considered spinal cord injury or spina bifida. Longstanding diabetes, extensive pelvic or back surgery, multiple sclerosis, or stroke can all have associated neurogenic changes to bladder function. Patients with neurogenic bladder have a markedly increased incidence of upper and lower tract UTI because of urinary stasis, frequent asymptomatic bacteriuria, bacterial seeding of the upper tracts due to reflux, as well as frequent instrumentation.[5] It is important to remember that asymptomatic bacteriuria is generally not treated in this population. However, these patients may not present with classic symptoms of cystitis or pyelonephritis due to their altered sensorium and abnormal voiding patterns. Instead of presenting with dysuria or flank pain, patients may present with complaints of increased urinary leakage, malodorous urine, fever, nonlocalizing abdominal or back pain, lethargy, or increased difficulty performing urethral catheterization.[5] UA and urine culture should be performed before the initiation of empiric antimicrobials. If there is suspicion of upper tract involvement, complete blood count and serum chemistry may also be informative. Upper tract imaging with ultrasound can assess for hydronephrosis, kidney or bladder calculi, bladder diverticula, and evidence of upper urinary tract deterioration (ie, parenchymal thinning) secondary to longstanding high urine storage and voiding pressures. If the patient is acutely ill at presentation, cross-sectional imaging with CT is indicated. In that setting, indwelling urethral catheter placement is prudent to maximize urinary drainage. If patients have urolithiasis or diverticulum on imaging or have not previously had urodynamic studies and regular follow-up with a urologist, urologic consultation should be performed. Urodynamic evaluation and cystoscopic interventions should be deferred until after resolution of acute illness. Patients may ultimately need changes made to their bladder management practices or operative interventions to reduce the risk of symptomatic infection.

Prostatitis

Prostatitis is one of the most common, yet challenging urologic problems in men of all ages. It is the most common urologic condition in men age less than 50 years and the third most common condition in men greater than 50, accounting for more than 2 million primary care and specialist visits annually.[16] Prostatitis encompasses 4 clinical entities: acute bacterial prostatitis, chronic bacterial prostatitis, chronic pelvic pain syndrome, and asymptomatic prostatitis.[17] Acute and chronic bacterial prostatitis are distinguished from the others in that a causative agent can be isolated on standard microbiological testing. For this reason, the scope of this work is limited to these 2 entities. Symptoms can range from those of acute systemic illness to persistent lower urinary tract symptoms, pelvic pain, and sexual dysfunction. Chronic symptoms can significantly alter both mental and physical quality of life in affected men.

Acute bacterial prostatitis

Acute prostatitis is an urgent, life-threatening clinical condition. The presentation is most commonly characterized by the rapid onset of fever, perineal and pelvic pain, and worsening obstructive and irritative voiding symptoms, often without a prodrome. Healthy, anatomically normal men can be affected if they acquire prostatic infection with a virulent microorganism. The key to proper management of this disease is timely recognition and intervention. Physical examination is perhaps the most important portion of the evaluation, but must be approached with care and caution. A gentle digital rectal examination will reveal a tender, boggy, prostate. Care must be taken to avoid a firm touch or overt prostatic massage, as this is thought to contribute to systemic seeding. In the setting of urinary retention, urethral catheterization should avoided in favor of suprapubic drainage established by a urologic practitioner, due to the friable nature of the prostate in this condition. The patient is often admitted for observation. Blood and urine cultures should be performed and empiric broad-spectrum antibiosis should be initiated soon thereafter. Gram-negative organisms are the most common causative agents, with E coli, Serratia, and Klebsiella being the most common isolates. Pseudomonas and gram-positive enterococci are more rare causes.[5] With proper intervention, complete resolution without long-term sequelae is likely. Only approximately 5% of patients with acute prostatitis develop chronic symptoms.[18]

Chronic bacterial prostatitis

Chronic bacterial prostatitis is characterized by persistent or relapsing and remitting pelvic pain and/or irritative voiding symptoms associated with the presence of bacteria localized to the prostate. Surprisingly, this entity represents only 5% to 15% of cases of prostatitis, because bacteria cannot be isolated in most cases. Most men with the diagnosis of prostatitis have the chronic, abacterial form and thus do not meet the criteria of complicated UTI. When encountered, these men should be referred to a urologist immediately in lieu of undertaking a trial of antimicrobial therapy because such therapy is unlikely to improve symptoms and increases the risk of development of infection with antimicrobial resistant pathogens.

Those with true chronic bacterial prostatitis often report a history of recurrent UTI, 25% to 43% cases in the literature.[19] Risk factors for the condition include urethral catheterization or instrumentation, dysfunctional voiding, condom catheter use, and unprotected anal intercourse.[20] Diagnosis is made by thorough history and physical examination, as well as specialized technique for obtaining UA and urine culture data. The first priority in obtaining history is to exclude more serious causes of irritative voiding symptoms including malignancy, sexually transmitted infection, and genitourinary anomalies. Any reported history of gross hematuria necessitates cystoscopic evaluation and cross-sectional imaging to evaluate for upper and lower tract cancers and stones. Detailed sexual history will reveal both contributory genital infections and related sexual dysfunction.

A thorough genital examination should be performed to assess for skin lesions, urethral discharge, scrotal lesions or pain, and prostatic tenderness and nodularity. The mandatory laboratory evaluation includes UA with microscopy, urine culture, and an assessment of postvoid residual urine volume. If these tests fail to be diagnostic of the condition, urologic consultation should be undertaken. A urologist can perform the gold-standard diagnostic evaluation, the "4-Glass Test." It is a localization culture consisting of 4 carefully timed specimens obtained from a single void, allowing for collection of samples that will be representative of bacterial milieu of the urethra, bladder, and 2 levels of prostatic secretions (pure expressed prostatic secretions and secretions admixed with the end of the voided urine). Each specimen is examined microscopically and by culture. A 10-fold increase in bacterial count in the specimen that contains prostatic secretions, when compared with those from the bladder or urethra, is diagnostic for chronic bacterial prostatitis.

The treatment of chronic bacterial prostatitis often involves culture-directed antimicrobial therapy. Fluroquinolones and trimethoprim sulfamethoxazole (TMP-SMX) are the most commonly used agents because of their good gram-negative coverage, low cost, and adequate prostate penetration. However, quinolones have been shown to exhibit a greater rate of bacterial eradication, with a markedly shorter course compared with TMP-SMX. A review of several clinical studies reveals that with a 4- to 6-week course of fluoroquinolones, bacterial eradication was achieved at a rate of 60% to 90%, whereas a 12-week course of TMP-SMX achieves cure only 30% to 50% of the time.[21]

When traditional antimicrobial therapy fails to eradicate infection, prophylactic antibiotic regimens can effectively reduce the number and frequency of symptomatic infections. Continuous, or symptom-dependent, "self-start" regimens can be tried. Continuous regimens consist of a single daily dose of antimicrobial directed at an identified bacterial isolate from the prostate. The dosing interval can be titrated to the greatest interval, which will still allow effective suppression. Titration should ideally be initiated within 6 months of starting the regimen, to minimize prolonged antimicrobial use as much as possible while maintaining symptoms relief. On a self-start regimen, men self-collect urine for culture and initiate antimicrobials at the onset of symptoms.

For patients whose symptoms are refractory to antibiotic therapy, radical transurethral resection of the colonized prostatic tissue has been advocated.

Genitourinary Instrumentation and Antimicrobial Prophylaxis

Genitourinary instrumentation is a significant risk factor for symptomatic upper and lower tract infections. Without antimicrobial prophylaxis, the incidence of UTI genitourinary instrumentation can be as high as 20%, depending on the procedure. Despite confirmation of negative preoperative urine culture, use of sterile technique, and perioperative antiobiosis, UTI after a variety urologic procedure ranges from 0.5% to 7%.[5] Although there is no consensus about periprocedure prophylaxis, many urologists routinely obtain preoperative urine cultures to decrease the risk of postoperative infections and help guide periprocedural antibiotic selection. The timing of culture before the surgery is a matter of individual practice, but the shorter the interval to surgery, the better, ideally within 1 to 2 weeks. This preoperative routine is feasible for planned procedures but may be challenging for urgent and emergent surgery. In these instances, urine can be obtained preoperatively for culture; empiric perioperative antimicrobials can be selected based on the most common uropathogens and continued until urine culture data are available. When culture data are unavailable or negative for microorganisms, cephalosporins, fluoroquinolones, and aminoglycosides are generally favored.

The American Urologic Association has published a best practice policy statement on antimicrobial prophylaxis for urologic surgery,[22] which is a valuable resource to help guide empiric antibiotic selection for various common urologic procedures. It recommends preoperative cultures and perioperative antibiosis for all procedures with moderate to high levels of manipulation in the genitourinary tract (ie, ureteroscopy, shockwave lithotripsy, open procedures). For procedures with a low level of manipulation, like catheter removal or flexible cystoscopy, prophylaxis is only recommended in compromised patients in whom infection may translate into undue morbidity (ie, immunosuppression, pregnancy).

Prostate Biopsy

Prostate needle biopsy deserves special consideration with regard to procedure prophylaxis because it is performed via a transrectal approach and thus facilitates translocation of bowel flora into the genitourinary tract. Before widespread use of antimicrobial prophylaxis for this procedure, the rate of infectious complications was reported as high as 37%. With routine prophylaxis, the current rate has been reduced to 2% to 6%, with a 0.5% to 1.5% incidence of sepsis.[23] The most widely used preprocedure protocol is urine culture with a full course of culture-directed therapy for all positives, and oral fluoroquinolone prophylaxis initiated 1 hour before the procedure and continued for 1 to 5 doses, 12 hours after the procedure.

However, in this era of widespread antimicrobial use, nearly one-quarter of men affected by postbiopsy infectious complications have been found to have fluoroquinolone-resistant isolates on postprocedure cultures, despite having negative urine cultures or fluoroquinolone-sensitive infections before biopsy,[24,25] which has led to exploration of the rectal flora as the reservoir for these isolates. Taylor and colleagues[26] performed preprocedure rectal swab cultures and found that 20% of men undergoing prostate biopsy at an urban, tertiary care center demonstrated ciprofloxacin-resistant organisms. Eighty-seven percent of these resistant isolates were *E coli*. When preprocedure prophylaxis targeted rectal isolates, the infectious complication rate was reduced to 0% compared with a 2.6% complication rate in the control arm receiving standard fluoroquinolone prophylaxis without rectal culture data. In addition, this reduction in complications translated into a 70% reduction in the hospital cost associated with performing preprocedure screening and prophylaxis.

SUMMARY

Complicated UTI can have diverse presentation and clinical course and thus often presents a diagnostic and therapeutic challenge for the treating physician. Timely recognition of complicated infections is the best method for optimizing therapeutic approach and minimizing patient morbidity and mortality. Being organized and informed in one's approach to the evaluation and treatment of individuals with known and suspected complicated UTI offers the best chance of providing optimal management. A complete medical history should illuminate patterns of infection and all risk factors, which may contribute to untoward outcomes or excessive morbidity. Timely and appropriate empiric therapy can halt conversion to serious systemic infection and improve symptoms, while the medical evaluation evolves. Having knowledge of which laboratory and imaging studies will be most informative in certain clinical scenarios will help facilitate timely urologic intervention when indicated.

REFERENCES

1. Foxman B. Epidemiology of urinary tract infection: incidence, morbidity and economic cost. Am J Med 2002;113(Supp 1A):5S–13S.

2. Schaeffer AJ, Schaeffer EM. Infections of the urinary tract. In: Wein AJ, Kavoussi LR, editors. Campbell-Walsh urology. 10th edition. Philadelphia: SaundersElservier; 2011. p. 258–326.
3. Eliakim-Raz N, Yahav D, Paul M, et al. Duration of antibiotic therapy for acute pyelonephritis and septic urinary tract infection. J Antimicrob Chemother 2013; 68(10):2183–91. http://dx.doi.org/10.1093/jac/dkt177.
4. Mazor-Dray E, Levy A, Schlaeffer F, et al. Maternal urinary tract infection: is it independently associated with adverse pregnancy outcome? J Matern Fetal Neonatal Med 2009;22(2):124–8.
5. Stamey TA. Pathogenesis and treatment of urinary tract infections. Baltimore (MD): Williams & Wilkins; 1980.
6. Smaill F, Vazquez JC. Antibiotics for asymptomatic bacteriuria in pregnancy. Cochrane Database Syst Rev 2007;(2):CD000490.
7. Whalley P. Bacteriuria of pregnancy. Am J Obstet Gynecol 1967;97(5):723–38.
8. Sweet RL. Bacteriuria and pyelonephritis during pregnancy. Semin Perinatol 1977;1(1):25–40.
9. Srirangam MJ, Hickerton B, VanCleynenbreugel B. Management of urinary calculi in pregnancy: a review. J Endourol 2008;22(5):867–75.
10. Norlin A, Lindell B, Granberg PO, et al. Urolithiasis: a study of its frequency. Scand J Urol Nephrol 1976;10:150–3.
11. Scales CD, Smith AC, Hanley JM, et al. Prevalence of kidney stones in the United States. Eur Urol 2012;62:160–5.
12. Levy FL, Adams-Huet B, Pak CY. Ambulatory evaluation of nephrolithiasis: an update from a 1980 protocol. Am J Med 1995;98:50–9.
13. Gardiner RA, Gwynne RA, Roberts SA. Perinephric abscess. BJU Int 2011; 107(Suppl 3):20–3.
14. Coelho RF, Schneider-Montiero ED, Mesquita JL. Renal and perinephric abscess: analysis of 65 consecutive cases. World J Surg 2007;31:431–6.
15. Cotran R. Experimental pyelonephritis. In: Rouiller C, Muller A, editors. The kidney. New York: Academic; 1969. p. 269–361.
16. McNaughton Collins M, Stafford RS, O'Leary MP. How common is prostatitis? A national survey of physical visits. J Urol 1998;51:578–84.
17. Litwin MS, McNaughton Collins M. The National Institutes of Health chronic prostatitis/chronic pelvic pain syndrome symptom index: development and validation of a new outcome measure. J Urol 1999;162(2):369–75.
18. Cho R, Lee KS, Jeon JS. Clinical outcome of acute prostatitis, a multicenter study. J Urol 2005;173(4):S28.
19. Weidner W, Ludwig M. Diagnostic management of chronic prostatitis. In: Weider W, Madsen PO, Schiefer HG, editors. Prostatitis—etiopathology, diagnosis and therapy. Berlin: Springer; 1994. p. 158–74.
20. Le B, Schaeffer AJ. Chronic prostatitis. Clin Evid (Online) 2011;07:1802.
21. Kurze E, Kaplan S. Cost effectiveness model comparing trimethoprimsulfamethoxazole and ciprofloxacin for treatment of chronic bacterial prostatitis. Eur Urol 2002;42(2):163–6.
22. Wolf S, Bennet CJ, Dmochowski RR, et al. Best practice policy statement on urologic surgery antimicrobial prophylaxis. J Urol 2008;179:1379–90.
23. Zani EL, Clark OA, Rodrigues Netto N Jr. Antibiotic prophylaxis for transrectal prostate biopsy. Cochrane Database Syst Rev 2011;(5):CD006576.
24. Zaytoun OM, Vargo EH, Rajan R, et al. Emergence of fluoroquinolone-resistant Escherichia coli as cause of postprostate biopsy infection: implications for prophylaxis and treatment. Urology 2011;77(5):1035–41.

25. Carignan A, Roussy JF, Lapointe V, et al. Increasing risk of infectious complications after transrectal ultrasound-guided prostate biopsies: time to reassess antimicrobial prophylaxis? Eur Urol 2012;62(3):453–9.
26. Taylor AK, Zembower TR, Nadler RB, et al. Targeted antimicrobial prophylaxis using rectal swab cultures in men undergoing transrectal ultrasound guided prostate biopsy is associated with reduced incidence of postoperative infectious complications and cost of care. J Urol 2012;187(4):1275–9.

Prevention of Recurrent Urinary Tract Infections in Women
Antimicrobial and Nonantimicrobial Strategies

Suzanne E. Geerlings, MD, PhD*, Mariëlle A.J. Beerepoot, MD, PhD,
Jan M. Prins, MD, PhD

KEYWORDS

- Recurrent urinary tract infections • Antimicrobial prophylaxis
- Non-antimicrobial strategies • Cranberries • Lactobacilli • Methenamine

KEY POINTS

- Recurrent urinary tract infections (UTIs) are common, especially in women.
- A differentiation must be made between persistence, relapse, and reinfection of the urinary tract. All recommendations concern patients with reinfections.
- In a persistent UTI, the cause must be evaluated. In a relapse of the UTI, the treatment can given for a longer period.
- Self-diagnosis and self-treatment of recurrences is reliable in premenopausal and postmenopausal women with recurrent UTIs.
- Methenamine hippurate can be used for a maximum of 1 week to prevent UTI in patients without urinary tract abnormalities.
- The use of ascorbic acid (vitamin C) is not recommended in the prevention of UTIs.
- In premenopausal women with recurrent UTIs, the following prophylaxis can be considered to decrease the number of recurrent episodes:
  ○ Daily or postcoital low-dose antimicrobial therapy
  ○ Cranberry products
  ○ *Lactobacillus crispatus* intravaginal suppository
- In postmenopausal women with recurrent UTIs, the following prophylaxis can be considered to decrease the number of recurrent episodes:
  ○ Daily or postcoital low-dose antimicrobial therapy
  ○ Topical estrogens
  ○ Oral capsules with *L rhamnosus* GR-1 and *L reuteri* RC-14

Division Infectious Diseases, Department of Internal Medicine, Academic Medical Center, Room F4-217, Meibergdreef 9, 1105 AZ Amsterdam, The Netherlands
* Corresponding author.
E-mail address: s.e.geerlings@amc.uva.nl

Infect Dis Clin N Am 28 (2014) 135–147
http://dx.doi.org/10.1016/j.idc.2013.10.001
0891-5520/14/$ – see front matter © 2014 Elsevier Inc. All rights reserved.
id.theclinics.com

INTRODUCTION

Urinary tract infections (UTIs) are common infections, especially in women. Recurrent UTIs are defined in the literature by 3 episodes of a UTI in the preceding 12 months or 2 episodes in the preceding 6 months. Approximately 50% to 70% of women have a UTI sometime during their lifetime and 20% to 30% of this group have recurrent UTIs.[1,2] In general, it is recommended to exclude anatomic or functional abnormalities of the urogenital tract as a cause of recurrent UTIs in men and postmenopausal women. In premenopausal women, the yield of most diagnostic procedures for this indication is low.[3]

There are 4 patterns of response of bacteriuria to therapy: cure, bacteriologic persistence, bacteriologic relapse, or reinfection. Bacteriologic persistence is persistence of bacteriuria with the same microorganism after 48 hours of treatment. Relapse (clinical and bacteriologic) is an infection with the same microorganism that caused the initial infection and usually occurs within 1 to 2 weeks after the cessation of treatment. A relapse indicates that the infecting organism has persisted in the urinary tract despite a good clinical response during treatment. Reinfection is an infection after sterilization of the urine. Most of the time another bacterial species is cultured. Both persistence and relapse may be related to inadequate treatment. Therefore, it is important to determine whether recurrent UTIs are relapses or reinfections and to make a differentiation between these patterns, because this has treatment consequences. Experts have the opinion that in a persistent UTI the cause must be evaluated. In a relapsed UTI, the treatment can be given for a longer period. This review only discusses the prevention of reinfections. Because women have the majority of recurrent UTIs, and recurrent UTIs in men might be considered chronic bacterial prostatitis, which is a different disease with different prevention and treatment strategies, the content of this article is limited to recurrent UTIs in women.

The first consideration in prevention of recurrent UTIs is to address modifiable behavioral practices. For example, urination after sexual intercourse in women is believed to decrease the incidence of UTIs. For some of these behavioral strategies, scientific evidence is missing, but they seem logical from a pathophysiologic point of view. Other effective strategies for the prevention of recurrent UTIs can be divided into antimicrobial or nonantimicrobial strategies.

ANTIMICROBIAL PROPHYLAXIS

Low-dose antimicrobial therapy remains an effective intervention to manage frequent, recurrent, acute uncomplicated UTI. The antimicrobial may be given as daily or every-other-day therapy, usually at bedtime, or as postcoital prophylaxis. Experts suggest an initial duration of prophylaxis of 6 months; however, 50% of women experience recurrence by 3 months after discontinuation of the prophylactic antimicrobial. When this occurs, prophylaxis may be reinstituted for 1 or 2 years.

A Cochrane review[1] included 19 studies involving 1120 women. During active prophylaxis, the rate range of microbiological recurrence per patient-year was 0 to 0.9 person-year in the antibiotic group versus 0.8 to 3.6 person-years with placebo. The relative risk (RR) of having 1 microbiological recurrence was 0.21 (95% CI, 0.13–0.34) favoring antibiotic, and the number needed to treat (NNT) was 1.85 women. For clinical recurrences, the RR was 0.15 (95% CI, 0.08–0.28) and the NNT was also 1.85 women. The RR of having 1 microbiological recurrence after prophylaxis was 0.82 (95% CI, 0.44–1.53). This Cochrane review, however, was published nearly 10 years ago and antimicrobial resistance has increased since then. Therefore, it is not clear whether the same effectiveness will be reached in the present day. The number of side effects was low[1]: RR for severe side effects was 1.58 (95% CI, 0.47–5.28) and for other side effects 1.78 (95% CI, 1.06–3.00), favoring placebo. Side effects included vaginal and oral candidiasis and gastrointestinal symptoms.[1] One randomized controlled trial (RCT) compared postcoital versus continuous daily ciprofloxacin and found no significant difference in rates of UTIs, suggesting that postcoital treatment could be offered to women who have UTI associated with sexual intercourse.[4]

In a more recent study, 317 women with recurrent UTIs were randomized to receive fosfomycin (3 g) trometamol equivalent or placebo every 10 days during 6 months. The incidence of UTIs was in favor of the fosfomycin, with an incidence of 0.14 infections/patient-year in the fosfomycin group and of 2.97 infections/patient-year in the placebo group (P<.001).[5]

In conclusion, low-dose daily or postcoital antimicrobial prophylaxis is effective in the prevention of recurrent UTIs.

SELF-DIAGNOSIS AND SELF-TREATMENT WITH ANTIMICROBIALS

Continuous prophylaxis may result in unnecessary antimicrobial use in women who have infrequent recurrences or clustered recurrences. An alternative strategy is patient self-diagnosis and self-treatment, which means that women start with antimicrobial treatment, which they already have at home, when they think that they have a UTI. This may decrease antimicrobial use and improve patient convenience.

In a prospective study, the accuracy of self-diagnosis and the cure rates seen with self-treatment (or patient-initiated therapy) of UTIs was determined in 172 women (mean age 23 years) who had a history of recurrent UTIs. A total number of 88 of 172 women self-diagnosed a total of 172 UTIs. Laboratory evaluation showed a uropathogen in 144 cases (84%), sterile pyuria in 19 cases (11%), and no pyuria or bacteriuria in 9 cases (5%). Clinical and microbiological cures occurred in 92% and 96%, respectively, of culture-confirmed episodes. No serious adverse events occurred.[2]

In a smaller study, 34 women (mean age 36 years) were enrolled. A total of 28 women followed for 355 months had 84 symptomatic episodes; 67 of 84 UTIs (80%) were confirmed microbiologically. Bacteriuria with symptoms of UTI was defined as significant if there were at least $10e2$ uropathogens per mL. Cure was defined as the resolution of symptoms (clinical) or no post-treatment bacteriuria (microbiological) at the 5- to 9-days' follow-up visit. Of the 84 symptomatic episodes, 78 (92%) responded clinically to self-treatment. Of the 78 cultured episodes, 11 (14%) were culture negative. No adverse effects occurred.[6]

Also, in older women, the concept of self-diagnosis and self-treatment was studied: 68 postmenopausal women were randomized to take a low-dose antibiotic each night (continuous group, n = 37) or a single-dose antibiotic each time they experienced symptoms predisposing to UTI (intermittent group, n = 31). During the 12-month study, patients experienced 1.4 and 1.9 UTIs per patient in the continuous and the intermittent groups, respectively, which was lower than the incidence of UTIs in the previous 12 months in these patients (4.7 and 5.1 UTIs per patient, respectively). The incidence of gastrointestinal adverse events was significantly lower in the intermittent group compared with the continuous group (9.1% vs 30.0%).[7]

In conclusion, women can self-diagnose and self-treat a recurrent UTI.

NONANTIMICROBIAL STRATEGIES

Antibiotics are the main driving force in the development of antibiotic resistance and can lead to resistance not only of the causative microorganisms but also of the commensal flora.[8,9] The increasing resistance rates of *Escherichia coli* isolates (the most prevalent uropathogen) to antimicrobial agents has stimulated interest in nonantibiotic methods for the prevention of UTIs. Studies evaluating vitamin C, cranberries, estrogens, lactobacilli, methenamine, and immunoprophylaxis are described.

Vitamin C (Ascorbic Acid)

Many women use vitamin C as a prevention method against UTI, but only 2 trials have been performed, with contradictory results.

In the first study, the effect of ascorbic acid on urine pH was studied in spinal cord injury patients. The study was designed to compare the baseline urine pH and after the administration of placebo or ascorbic acid (500 mg 4 times daily). A total of 38 patients began the study, but only 13 patients completed the study. A significant decrease in urine pH value was not obtained. There was no clinical benefit from the use of ascorbic acid; 2 patients in the ascorbic acid and 1 patient in the placebo group developed a UTI between the sixth and eighth days after start.[10]

In the other nonrandomized trial in pregnant women, it was shown that daily intake of a vitamin regimen with ascorbic acid (100 mg for 3 months) reduced the incidence of UTIs by 30% compared with a vitamin regimen without acorbic acid.[11] It is difficult to understand, however, the results of this trial, because the daily vitamin C dose was very low and the endpoint of symptoms of a UTI were subjective without microbiological confirmation.

In conclusion, use of ascorbic acid (vitamin C) cannot be recommended for the prevention of UTIs based on currently available evidence.

Cranberries

Cranberries have been used in the prevention of UTIs for many years. The mechanism of action has not been completely elucidated, but cranberries contain type A proanthocyanidins (PACs), which can inhibit the adherence of P fimbriae of *E coli* to the uroepithelial cell receptors.[12]

Several studies have been performed that compared cranberry products to placebo or no treatment. Kontiokari and colleagues[13] showed that the probability of remaining UTI-free was lower in patients treated with cranberry-lingonberry juice compared with the lactobacillus and control groups. After 6 months, 8 (16%) of the women in the cranberry group, 19 (38%) in the lactobacillus group, and 18 (36%) in the control group had at least 1 UTI (log rank, $P = .023$). The intervention with cranberry-lingonberry juice was stopped prematurely after 6 months because the manufacturer stopped producing the juice. The difference remained significant, however, 6 months after stopping the cranberry prophylaxis. There were occasional complaints about the bitter taste of the cranberry juice.[13]

Stothers[14] compared cranberry juice as well as cranberry tablets to placebo. In this double-blind, double-dummy study, women were randomized to 1 of 3 groups: placebo juice and placebo tablets, placebo juice and cranberry tablets, and cranberry juice and placebo tablets. Tablets were taken twice and juice (250 mL) 3 times daily. In these, studies cranberry products reduced UTI recurrences (RR 0.53; 95% CI, 0.33–0.83) and significantly decreased the proportion of women experiencing at least 1 symptomatic UTI during the 12-months of follow-up. These proportions were 20% in the cranberry tablets and 18% in the cranberry juice group compared with 32% in the placebo group.

Considering the side effects, 3 women (6%) receiving cranberry juice reported reflux; 2 of them dropped out of the study due to this problem. Ten women (20%) in the cranberry tablet group had complaints about the size of the tablets, but this did not lead to withdrawal. In addition, 4 women (8%) experienced mild nausea. These studies are the

2 main studies in healthy adult women with recurrent UTIs that were included in a Cochrane review.[15] In contrast to the recent update, this older Cochrane review[15] included 10 studies (n = 1049; 5 crossover and 5 parallel groups) with only patients with recurrent UTIs. Cranberry/cranberry-lingonberry juice versus placebo was evaluated in 7 studies, and cranberry tablets versus placebo in 4 studies (1 study evaluated both juice and tablets). Cranberry products significantly reduced the incidence of UTIs at 12 months (RR 0.65; 95% CI, 0.46–0.90) compared with placebo/control.

Cranberry products were more effective in reducing the incidence of UTIs in women with recurrent UTIs than in elderly men and women or people requiring catheterization. The investigators concluded that there is some evidence that cranberry juice may decrease the number of symptomatic UTIs over a 12-month period, particularly for women with recurrent UTIs. Its effectiveness for other groups is less certain. The large number of dropouts/withdrawals indicates that cranberry juice may not be acceptable over long periods of time and the optimum dosage or method of administration (eg, juice, tablets, or capsules) is not clear. Finally, daily cranberry products (juice or tablets) decrease the frequency of recurrent infection by approximately 30% to 40% compared with 90% to 95% effectiveness of antimicrobial use.[15]

Barbosa-Cesnik and colleagues[16] investigated in a double-blind, placebo-controlled trial the effects of cranberry on risk of recurring UTIs among 319 college women presenting with an acute UTI. Participants were followed-up until a second UTI or for 6 months. Overall, the recurrence rate was 16.9% (95% CI, 12.8%–21.0%), and the distribution of the recurrences was similar between study groups, with the active cranberry group presenting a slightly higher recurrence rate (20.0% vs 14.0%). The presence of urinary symptoms at 3 days, 1 to 2 weeks, and at greater than or equal to 1 month was similar between study groups, with overall no marked differences. The study population, however, consisted of women with at least 1 UTI instead of recurrent UTIs.

In 2 studies the effectiveness of cranberry extract was compared with low-dose antibiotics (standard prophylaxis).[8,17] In the first study,[17] 137 older women with 2 or more antibiotic-treated UTIs in the previous 12 months were randomized to receive either cranberry extract (500 mg) or trimethoprim (TMP) (100 mg) for 6 months: 39 of 137 participants (28%) had an antibiotic-treated UTI (25 in the cranberry group and 14 in the TMP group) (RR 1.616; 95% CI, 0.93–2.79; P = .08). The time to first recurrence of UTI was not significantly different between the groups (P = .10). The median time to recurrence of UTI was 84.5 days in the cranberry group and 91 days in the TMP group (P = .479); 6 of 69 women (9%) from the cranberry group and 11 of 68 women (16%) from the TMP group withdrew (P = .205). The investigators conclude that TMP had a limited advantage over cranberry extract in the prevention of recurrent UTIs in older women.

In another study of a similar population of women with at least 1 previous UTI and using the same active and placebo juices, there was a nonsignificant reduction in the time of UTI in the cranberry group compared with the placebo group. The adjusted hazard ratio for UTI in the cranberry juice group versus the placebo group was 0.68 (95% CI, 0.33–1.39; P = .29). The proportion of women with P-fimbriated urinary *E coli* isolates during the intervention phase was 10 of 23 (43.5%) in the cranberry juice group and 8 of 10 (80.0%) in the placebo group (P = .07), consistent with the postulated mechanism of cranberry products reducing adherence of P-fimbriated *E coli* to the bladder.[18]

A more recent study showed that cranberry capsules are less effective than low-dose (480 mg) TMP–sulfamethoxazole(SMX) in the prevention of recurrent UTIs in premenopausal women. In contrast to low-dose TMP-SMX, however, cranberries did not result into in an increase in resistant microorganisms in the commensal flora.[8]

In conclusion, the cranberry products studied decreased the frequency of recurrent infection by approximately 30% to 40% in women with recurrent UTIs but are less effective compared with low-dose antimicrobial prophylaxis. The optimal dose of cranberry product has still to be determined, however.

Estrogens

Estrogen replacement restores atrophic mucosa, lowers vaginal pH, and may prevent UTIs. In a Cochrane review, 9 studies (3345 women) with estrogens were included.[19] Oral estrogens did not reduce UTI compared with placebo (4 studies, 2798 women: RR 1.08; 95% CI, 0.88–1.33). In addition, oral estrogens were found associated with coronary heart disease, venous thromboembolism, stroke, and breast cancer. Therefore, oral estrogens are no longer recommended in postmenopausal women to prevent recurrent UTIs.

Compared with placebo, vaginal estrogens reduced the number of UTIs in 2 small studies using different application methods. The RRs for UTI were 0.25 (95% CI, 0.13–0.50)[20] and 0.64 (95% CI, 0.47–0.86), respectively.[21] Adverse events for vaginal estrogens were breast tenderness, vaginal bleeding or spotting, nonphysiologic discharge, vaginal irritation, burning, and itching.

In another study, the efficacy and safety of an estriol-containing vaginal pessary was compared with the use of oral nitrofurantoin therapy in postmenopausal women with recurrent UTIs. Over a period of 9 months, 86 women received an estriol-containing vaginal pessary (0.5 mg estriol) twice weekly, and 85 women received nitrofurantoin (100 mg) once daily: 124 episodes of UTI were recorded in women who received estriol-releasing pessaries and 48 episodes in women treated with nitrofurantoin ($P = .0003$); 28 women (32.6%) who received estriol had no episodes of UTI versus 41 women (48.2%).[22]

In conclusion, vaginal, but not oral, estrogens reduce the number of UTIs compared with placebo.

Lactobacilli

Specific lactobacilli strains have the ability to interfere with the adherence, growth, and colonization of the urogenital human epithelium by uropathogenic bacteria. This interaction is believed important in the maintenance of a normal urogenital flora and in the prevention of urogenital infection in women.[23] The use of probiotics to re-establish vaginal colonization with H_2O_2-producing lactobacilli has been investigated.

Studies have been performed with different strains of lactobacilli. In a study by Baerheim and colleagues,[24] 48 women were randomized to vaginal suppositories containing *L casei v rhamnosus*, twice weekly for 26 weeks, or placebo. The study from Kontiokari and colleagues[13] (discussed previously) was an open randomized trial in 150 women who had UTI caused by *E coli*. After being treated with antimicrobial agents for the UTI, they were randomly allocated to 1 of 3 groups. The first group received cranberry-lingonberry juice (50 mL per day), the second group took a *Lactobacillus* GG (100 mL; 4×10^{10} colony-forming units) drink 5 days per week, and a third group received no further treatment. In both studies,[13,24] lactobacilli prophylaxis did not show an advantage in terms of UTI prevention compared with placebo or no treatment. Baerheim and colleageus[24] reported a monthly incidence of symptomatic UTI of 0.21 in the *L casei* group and of 0.15 in the placebo group (incidence rate ratio 1.41; 95% CI, 0.88–1.98). Kontiokari and colleagues[13] did also not show a difference between *Lactobacillus* GG drink and no treatment. The numbers of women who had a UTI at 12 months were 21 (42.9%) and 19 (38.0%) in the lactobacillus and control groups, respectively. The mean number of UTIs experienced during the 12-month follow-up was 0.80 UTIs/patient in the lactobacilli-treated women compared with 0.76 UTI/patient in the control group.

Women using the *Lactobacillus* GG drink did not experience side effects.[13] In the study by Baerheim and colleagues,[24] in which women used vaginal suppositories, the most commonly reported adverse reaction (in 16% of women) was vaginal discharge after taking the suppositories.

A more recent double-blind, placebo-controlled trial studied *L crispatus*–containing intravaginal suppositories (Lactin-V) (daily for 5 days, then once weekly for 10 weeks). A total of 100 premenopausal women with at least 1 prior UTI in the preceding 12 months (median number lifetime UTIs 4.5) were randomized to receive either Lactin-V or placebo after treatment with antimicrobial agents for an acute UTI. Recurrent UTIs occurred in 7 of 48 women (15%) receiving Lactin-V compared with 13 of 48 women (27%) receiving placebo (RR 0.5; 95% CI, 0.2–1.2). High-level vaginal colonization with *L crispatus* ($\geq$10e6 throughout follow-up) was associated with a significant reduction in recurrent UTIs only for Lactin-V (RR for Lactin-V 0.07; RR for placebo 1.1; $P<.01$).[25]

In another RCT, 252 postmenopausal women with recurrent UTIs were randomized to receive 12 months of prophylaxis with TMP-SMX (480 mg once daily) or oral capsules containing 10e9 colony-forming units of *L rhamnosus* GR-1 and *L reuteri* RC-14 twice daily. The mean number of symptomatic UTIs in the year preceding randomization was 7.0 in the TMP-SMX group and 6.8 in the lactobacilli group. In the intention-to-treat analysis, after 12 months of prophylaxis, these numbers were 2.9 and 3.3, respectively. The between-treatment difference of 0.4 UTIs per year (95% CI, −0.4 to 1.5) was outside the noninferiority margin of 10% (**Fig. 1**). At least 1 symptomatic UTI occurred in 69.3% and 79.1% of the TMP-SMX and lactobacilli participants, respectively; median times to the first UTI were 6 and 3 months, respectively (log rank $P = .02$). After 1 month of TMP-SMX prophylaxis, however, resistance to TMP-SMX, TMP, and amoxicillin had increased from approximately 20% to 40% to approximately 80% to 95% in *E coli* from the feces and urine of asymptomatic women and among *E coli* causing a UTI. During the 3 months after TMP-SMX discontinuation, resistance levels gradually decreased. Resistance did not increase during lactobacilli prophylaxis.[9]

In conclusion, different lactobacilli strains show different results in the prevention of recurrent UTIs. The results with *L crispatus* intravaginal suppositories or oral capsules with *L rhamnosus* GR-1 and *L reuteri* RC-14 are promising.

Methenamine Salts

Methenamine salts act via the production of formaldehyde from hexamine, which acts as a bacteriostatic agent without affecting bacterial susceptibility. They are well tolerated. In vitro and in vivo studies suggest that a urinary pH below 5.5 is needed for bacteriostatic concentrations of free formaldehyde to be generated from methenamine hippurate. Therefore, UTIs with urease-producing *Proteus* (and possibly *Pseudomonas*), which increases urine pH through hydrolyzation of urea to ammonia, will not be prevented by methenamine due to insufficient generation of formaldehyde. Acidification of urine may be achieved with additional high doses of vitamin C (1–4 g). A Cochrane review included 13 studies (2032 participants) of methenamine hippurate.[26] Subgroup analyses suggested that methenamine hippurate may have some benefit in patients without urinary tract abnormalities or urinary catheters (symptomatic UTI—RR 0.24; 95% CI, 0.07–0.89; bacteriuria—RR 0.56; 95% CI, 0.37–0.83) but not in patients with known urinary tract abnormalities (symptomatic UTI—RR 1.54; 95% CI, 0.38–6.20; bacteriuria—RR 1.29; 95% CI, 0.54–3.07). For short-term treatment

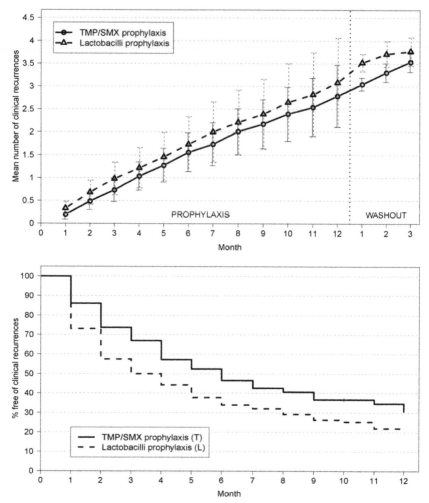

Fig. 1. Mean number of clinical recurrences during and after prophylaxis (*upper panel*) and time to first clinical recurrence (*lower panel*). Note: In the washout period, CIs are smaller because it represents data from all patients in the 3 months after discontinuation of the study medication, including those who had prematurely discontinued the study medication.

duration (1 week or less), there was a significant reduction in symptomatic UTIs in those without urinary tract abnormalities (RR 0.14; 95% CI, 0.05–0.38). The rate of adverse events was low.

In 2011, however, formaldehyde was officially declared carcinogenic by the National Toxicology Program. The exposure in the bladder to formaldehyde can be high if it is used at high doses for a prolonged time, but the risk of bladder cancer from use of methenamine is a theoretic risk, which has not been confirmed (National Toxicology Program, Department of Health and Human Services Report on Carcinogens, Twelfth Edition [2011] Formaldehyde).[27]

In conclusion, methenamine hippurate can be used for 1 week to prevent UTI in patients without urinary tract abnormalities. In the authors' opinion, methenamine hippurate can be used safely for a maximum of 1 week. Further studies, however, are needed.

Immunoactive Prophylaxis

Various bacterial extracts have been used in the management of recurrent UTIs. Experts mean that an effective bacterial extract must be able to stimulate the host's immune system to produce antibodies and cytokines.[28] The exact mechanisms of protection and immunologic basis are, however, still unclear.

Oral immunostimulant OM-89

The oral immunostimulant, OM-89, an extract of 18 different serotypes of heat-killed uropathogenic *E coli,* stimulates innate immunity by increasing neutrophils macrophage phagocytosis and via the upregulation of dendritic cells.

Four placebo-controlled studies,[29–32] with a total of 891 patients with recurrent UTIs, dealing with the oral immunostimulant OM-89 have been performed. During the intervention period, women had to use 1 capsule daily. The risk ratio for developing at least 1 UTI was significantly lower in the active treatment group (RR 0.61; 95% CI, 0.48–0.78) and the mean number of UTIs was approximately half compared with placebo.

The proportion of patients experiencing adverse events in the OM-89 groups was comparable to that in the placebo groups. Up to 13% of adverse events were considered treatment related. Headache and gastrointestinal complaints were reported most.

Vaginal vaccine Urovac

Urovac is a vaginal vaccine that contains 10 heat-killed uropathogenic bacterial species, including 6 different serotypes of uropathogenic *E coli*, *Proteus vulgaris*, *Klebsiella pneumoniae*, *Morganella morganii*, and *Enterococcus faecalis*. This vaccine induces primarily immunoglobulin G and immunoglobulin A in the urogenital tract, thereby reducing potential colonization of the vagina and bladder with uropathogens.[33] In 3 trials comprising 220 women,[33–35] all 3 performed by the same group of investigators, placebo was compared with primary immunization[34] or with primary immunization with booster immunizations.[33,35] Primary immunization consisted of 3 vaginal vaccine suppositories at weekly intervals (low-dose 1 vaccine dose and high-dose 2 vaccine doses per suppository). Booster immunization consisted of 3 additional vaccine suppositories at monthly intervals.

In 1 study,[34] no difference was found in the interval until first reinfection with the low-dose or high-dose vaginal vaccine. Therefore, results of both doses were combined for analysis of vaccine efficacy. The mean number of UTIs over the entire 20-week trial period was 1.4 in the vaccine and placebo-treated group. Similarly, no significant difference was seen in the proportion of women with at least 1 UTI ($P = .48$). When the analysis was restricted to the first 4 weeks of the study and to women who were off antibiotic prophylaxis, however, only 9% of the women in the treatment group had a UTI compared with 47% in the placebo group ($P = .003$). Also the time to first reinfection was longer (13 weeks) in the immunized patients compared with the control (8.7 weeks) patients ($P = .45$).

In 2 smaller studies[33,35] of the vaginal vaccine, the addition of booster vaccinations after the primary vaccination was evaluated. One vaccine dose consisted of 1×10^9 killed organisms[33] or 2×10^9 killed organisms.[35] Patients discontinued antibiotic prophylaxis before study enrollment. In the study from Uehling and colleagues,[35] the time until first reinfection and the proportion of women experiencing a UTI were both in favor of the booster immunization group compared with those receiving placebo or primary immunization only. Also, the mean number of UTIs during the follow-up of 6 months was lower in the women receiving booster immunization (1.1 UTIs) compared with those in women treated with placebo (1.5 UTIs) and primary immunization only (1.7 UTIs). Hopkins and colleagues[33] found similar results, placebo and primary immunization only were inferior to primary immunization with boosters.

In all studies using the vaginal vaccine, some women experienced vaginal irritation shortly after suppository insertions (4.9%–27.8%).

In conclusion, the results of the immunoactive prophylaxis with various bacterial extracts, especially the oral immunostimulant OM-89, seem promising, but the working mechanism must be more elucidated before this form can be introduced in clinical practice.

DISCUSSION

In patients with recurrent UTIs, a differentiation must be made between persistence, relapse, and reinfection. When a patient has a persistent UTI, the cause of this persistence must be evaluated (for example, for the presence of a stone or other nidus).

Considering recurrent UTIs or reinfections, the results of these studies show that low-dose antimicrobial prophylaxis is the most effective method to prevent recurrent UTIs. This results, however, in increasing resistance of uropathogenic bacteria and the commensal flora. The recently updated IDSA guideline on the treatment of uncomplicated UTI recommends taking into account this "collateral damage"[36] when prescribing antibiotics. Furthermore, it has been shown that different antimicrobial agents have different effects. In 1 study, the gram-negative aerobic flora was strongly affected during the administration of norfloxacin and TMP-SMX but not during nitrofurantoin.[37] These findings help in the selection of the most appropriate antimicrobial agent for prophylaxis of recurrent UTIs.

Concerning the use of vitamin C, it is difficult to understand the positive effect of the prevention trial in pregnant women, because the daily vitamin C dose was much lower (1×100 mg instead of 4×500 mg) than in the trial with the negative results. Moreover, the trial was not blinded and the endpoint was highly subjective.[11] Therefore, prophylaxis with vitamin C cannot be recommended. Vaginal estrogens are already used for many years worldwide. Vaginal irritation occurs frequently, however, and affects adherence.

Both cranberry juice and tablets reduced the occurrence of UTIs compared with placebo. In earlier studies, the chemical composition of available cranberry products was not standardized nor was the description of the dose. In addition, the bioequivalence between the juice and capsules or tablets is not clear. These factors make it difficult to compare studies and draw conclusions[15] (NCT00100061 2004). Therefore, the greatest challenge in the field of cranberry research is to determine the optimum dose of PACs to prevent UTIs in vivo. In 2010, Howell and colleagues[12] concluded, based on an ex vivo study in urine samples of volunteers who consumed cranberry powder, that PAC (72 mg per day) might offer some protection against bacterial adhesion and virulence in the urinary tract. The results of the dose-finding study (NCT00100061 2004) with cranberry products currently under way will determine the optimal dose for future cranberry product trials.

Prophylaxis with nonantimicrobial agents does not result in an increase of antimicrobial resistance of the commensal flora.[8,9] Therefore, the use of cranberry prophylaxis or intravaginal *L crispatus* intravaginal in premenopausal women and oral capsules with *L rhamnosus* GR-1 and *L reuteri* RC-14 or topical vaginal estrogen in postmenopausal women can be considered.

Among the different forms of immunoprophylaxis studied, the oral immunostimulant OM-89 seems the most promising to prevent recurrent UTIs. The results of a study comparing OM-89 with antibiotic prophylaxis in adults with recurrent UTIs are expected in the near future (https://www.clinicaltrialsregister.eu/ctr-search/trial/2007-004586-17/AT). Although there was a significant decrease in UTI recurrence with the vaginal vaccine, Urovac, the pooled finding for this nonantibiotic form of prophylaxis is based on a few studies. Therefore, confirmation by larger studies, by independent investigators, is necessary.

Due to the increasing resistance percentages of the causative microorganisms, it seems that more studies with nonantibiotic prophylaxis in the prevention of recurrent UTIs are warranted. Up to now, only a few studies have been undertaken that compared nonantibiotic prophylaxis with antibiotic prophylaxis to prevent recurrent UTIs.[8,9,17,22] Advantages other than simply reducing the rate of recurrent UTIs, such as reduced rates of development of antibiotic-resistant microbial flora that have been demonstrated with nonantimicrobial prevention strategies, need to be considered on an individual patient level.[9,38]

To optimally inform clinical decision making, head-to-head trials should be performed comparing the different forms of nonantibiotic prophylaxis with each other, with placebo, and/or with antibiotic prophylaxis, which still is the standard of care. In particular, the lactobacilli strains (oral and vaginal) and the oral immunostimulant OM-89 seem promising.

REFERENCES

1. Albert X, Huertas I, Pereiro II, et al. Antibiotics for preventing recurrent urinary tract infection in non-pregnant women. Cochrane Database Syst Rev 2004;(3): CD001209.
2. Gupta K, Hooton TM, Roberts PL, et al. Patient-initiated treatment of uncomplicated recurrent urinary tract infections in young women. Ann Intern Med 2001; 135(1):9–16.
3. van Haarst EP, van AG, Heldeweg EA, et al. Evaluation of the diagnostic workup in young women referred for recurrent lower urinary tract infections. Urology 2001;57(6):1068–72.
4. Melekos MD, Asbach HW, Gerharz E, et al. Post-intercourse versus daily ciprofloxacin prophylaxis for recurrent urinary tract infections in premenopausal women. J Urol 1997;157(3):935–9.
5. Rudenko N, Dorofeyev A. Prevention of recurrent lower urinary tract infections by long-term administration of fosfomycin trometamol. Double blind, randomized, parallel group, placebo controlled study. Arzneimittelforschung 2005;55(7):420–7.
6. Schaeffer AJ, Stuppy BA. Efficacy and safety of self-start therapy in women with recurrent urinary tract infections. J Urol 1999;161(1):207–11.
7. Zhong YH, Fang Y, Zhou JZ, et al. Effectiveness and safety of patientinitiated single-dose versus continuous low-dose antibiotic prophylaxis for recurrent urinary tract infections in postmenopausal women: a randomized controlled study. J Int Med Res 2011;39(6):2335–43.
8. Beerepoot MA, ter RG, Nys S, et al. Cranberries vs antibiotics to prevent urinary tract infections: a randomized double-blind noninferiority trial in premenopausal women. Arch Intern Med 2011;171(14):1270–8.
9. Beerepoot MA, ter RG, Nys S, et al. Lactobacilli vs antibiotics to prevent urinary tract infections: a randomized, double-blind, noninferiority trial in postmenopausal women. Arch Intern Med 2012;172(9):704–12.
10. Castello T, Girona L, Gomez MR, et al. The possible value of ascorbic acid as a prophylactic agent for urinary tract infection. Spinal Cord 1996;34(10):592–3.

11. Ochoa-Brust GJ, Fernandez AR, Villanueva-Ruiz GJ, et al. Daily intake of 100 mg ascorbic acid as urinary tract infection prophylactic agent during pregnancy. Acta Obstet Gynecol Scand 2007;86(7):783–7.

12. Howell AB, Botto H, Combescure C, et al. Dosage effect on uropathogenic Escherichia coli anti-adhesion activity in urine following consumption of cranberry powder standardized for proanthocyanidin content: a multicentric randomized double blind study. BMC Infect Dis 2010;10:94.

13. Kontiokari T, Sundqvist K, Nuutinen M, et al. Randomised trial of cranberry-lingonberry juice and Lactobacillus GG drink for the prevention of urinary tract infections in women. BMJ 2001;322(7302):1571.

14. Stothers L. A randomized trial to evaluate effectiveness and cost effectiveness of naturopathic cranberry products as prophylaxis against urinary tract infection in women. Can J Urol 2002;9(3):1558–62.

15. Jepson RG, Craig JC. Cranberries for preventing urinary tract infections. Cochrane Database Syst Rev 2008;(1):CD001321.

16. Barbosa-Cesnik C, Brown MB, Buxton M, et al. Cranberry juice fails to prevent recurrent urinary tract infection: results from a randomized placebo-controlled trial. Clin Infect Dis 2011;52(1):23–30.

17. McMurdo ME, Argo I, Phillips G, et al. Cranberry or trimethoprim for the prevention of recurrent urinary tract infections? A randomized controlled trial in older women. J Antimicrob Chemother 2009;63(2):389–95.

18. Stapleton AE, Dziura J, Hooton TM, et al. Recurrent urinary tract infection and urinary Escherichia coli in women ingesting cranberry juice daily: a randomized controlled trial. Mayo Clin Proc 2012;87(2):143–50.

19. Perrotta C, Aznar M, Mejia R, et al. Oestrogens for preventing recurrent urinary tract infection in postmenopausal women. Cochrane Database Syst Rev 2008;(2): CD005131.

20. Raz R, Stamm WE. A controlled trial of intravaginal estriol in postmenopausal women with recurrent urinary tract infections. N Engl J Med 1993;329(11):753–6.

21. Eriksen B. A randomized, open, parallel-group study on the preventive effect of an estradiol-releasing vaginal ring (Estring) on recurrent urinary tract infections in postmenopausal women. Am J Obstet Gynecol 1999;180(5):1072–9.

22. Raz R, Colodner R, Rohana Y, et al. Effectiveness of estriol-containing vaginal pessaries and nitrofurantoin macrocrystal therapy in the prevention of recurrent urinary tract infection in postmenopausal women. Clin Infect Dis 2003;36(11): 1362–8.

23. Falagas ME, Betsi GI, Tokas T, et al. Probiotics for prevention of recurrent urinary tract infections in women: a review of the evidence from microbiological and clinical studies. Drugs 2006;66(9):1253–61.

24. Baerheim A, Larsen E, Digranes A. Vaginal application of lactobacilli in the prophylaxis of recurrent lower urinary tract infection in women. Scand J Prim Health Care 1994;12(4):239–43.

25. Stapleton AE, Au-Yeung M, Hooton TM, et al. Randomized, placebo-controlled phase 2 trial of a Lactobacillus crispatus probiotic given intravaginally for prevention of recurrent urinary tract infection. Clin Infect Dis 2011;52(10):1212–7.

26. Lee BB, Simpson JM, Craig JC, et al. Methenamine hippurate for preventing urinary tract infections. Cochrane Database Syst Rev 2007;(4):CD003265.

27. Lee BS, Bhuta T, Simpson JM, et al. Methenamine hippurate for preventing urinary tract infections. Cochrane Database Syst Rev 2012;(10):CD003265.

28. Naber KG, Cho YH, Matsumoto T, et al. Immunoactive prophylaxis of recurrent urinary tract infections: a meta-analysis. Int J Antimicrob Agents 2009;33(2):111–9.

29. Tammen H. Immunobiotherapy with Uro-Vaxom in recurrent urinary tract infection. The German Urinary Tract Infection Study Group. Br J Urol 1990;65(1):6–9.
30. Schulman CC, Corbusier A, Michiels H, et al. Oral immunotherapy of recurrent urinary tract infections: a double-blind placebo-controlled multicenter study. J Urol 1993;150(3):917–21.
31. Magasi P, Panovics J, Illes A, et al. Uro-Vaxom and the management of recurrent urinary tract infection in adults: a randomized multicenter double-blind trial. Eur Urol 1994;26(2):137–40.
32. Bauer HW, Alloussi S, Egger G, et al. A long-term, multicenter, double-blind study of an Escherichia coli extract (OM-89) in female patients with recurrent urinary tract infections. Eur Urol 2005;47(4):542–8.
33. Hopkins WJ, Elkahwaji J, Beierle LM, et al. Vaginal mucosal vaccine for recurrent urinary tract infections in women: results of a phase 2 clinical trial. J Urol 2007; 177(4):1349–53.
34. Uehling DT, Hopkins WJ, Balish E, et al. Vaginal mucosal immunization for recurrent urinary tract infection: phase II clinical trial. J Urol 1997;157(6):2049–52.
35. Uehling DT, Hopkins WJ, Elkahwaji JE, et al. Phase 2 clinical trial of a vaginal mucosal vaccine for urinary tract infections. J Urol 2003;170(3):867–9.
36. Gupta K, Hooton TM, Naber KG, et al. International clinical practice guidelines for the treatment of acute uncomplicated cystitis and pyelonephritis in women: a 2010 update by the Infectious Diseases Society of America and the European Society for Microbiology and Infectious Diseases. Clin Infect Dis 2011;52(5): e103–20.
37. Mavromanolakis E, Maraki S, Samonis G, et al. Effect of norfloxacin, trimethoprim-sulfamethoxazole and nitrofurantoin on fecal flora of women with recurrent urinary tract infections. J Chemother 1997;9(3):203–7.
38. Trautner BW, Gupta K. The advantages of second best: comment on "Lactobacilli vs antibiotics to prevent urinary tract infections". Arch Intern Med 2012;172(9): 712–4.

Urinary Tract Infection Pathogenesis: Host Factors

Ann E. Stapleton, MD[a,b,*]

KEYWORDS

- Modifiable host factors • Nonmodifiable host factors • Sexual intercourse
- Estrogen status • Urogenital microbiota • Female gender

KEY POINTS

- Host factors in urinary tract infection include both modifiable aspects that patients and physicians may be able to influence and thus reduce risk, and nonmodifiable factors with future potential for therapeutics or risk profiling.
- Examples of modifiable host factors include sexual intercourse, choice of contraceptives, exposure to antimicrobials, estrogen status, and influences on the urogenital microbiota.
- Examples of nonmodifiable host factors include female gender and genetic influences.
- To assist patients in reducing the risk of UTI, currently clinicians should consider reviewing modifiable host factors and helping patients decide if relevant interventions are appropriate.
- In the future, genetically based, nonmodifiable host factors in the pathogenesis of UTI may be clinically relevant to risk profiling in certain populations, such as children.

INTRODUCTION

Epidemiology

Urinary tract infections (UTIs) are among the most common infections throughout the life span in both genders, in both ambulatory and hospitalized patients. Although the Centers for Disease Control and Prevention (CDC) do not designate UTI as a reportable disease, ambulatory visits for UTI are captured in the CDC annual National Ambulatory Medical Care Survey (NHAMCS).[1] According to most recent available data from the NHAMCS, in 2007 there were 8.6 million ambulatory visits for UTI in both men and

[a] Division of Allergy and Infectious Diseases, Medicine, Institute of Translational Health Sciences, University of Washington, Box 356423, Room BB1233, 1959 Northeast Pacific Street, Seattle, WA 98195, USA; [b] Clinical Research Center, Institute of Translational Health Sciences, University of Washington, 7 South UWMC, Box 356178, 1959 Northeast Pacific Street, Seattle, WA 98195, USA
* Division of Allergy and Infectious Diseases, Medicine, Institute of Translational Health Sciences, University of Washington, Box 356423, Room BB1233, 1959 Northeast Pacific Street, Seattle, WA 98195.
E-mail address: stapl@uw.edu

Infect Dis Clin N Am 28 (2014) 149–159
http://dx.doi.org/10.1016/j.idc.2013.10.006 **id.theclinics.com**
0891-5520/14/$ – see front matter © 2014 Elsevier Inc. All rights reserved.

women in the United States.[1] As described in greater detail herein, girls and women are disproportionately affected by UTI.[2]

Disease Description

Several specific syndromes of UTI are known, such as acute uncomplicated cystitis (AUC), or bladder infection, and acute uncomplicated pyelonephritis (AUP). AUC is defined as a compatible clinical syndrome, including symptoms such as dysuria, urinary frequency, or urgency occurring in an otherwise healthy, nonpregnant woman.[3] If laboratory studies are obtained, diagnostic findings include the presence of pyuria in voided urine and a urine culture positive for a uropathogen in amounts of at least 10^3 cfu/mL.[3] Clinically, AUP is characterized by fever, costovertebral angle tenderness, and/or flank pain, and other systemic symptoms, also in a nonpregnant, otherwise healthy woman, and the syndrome may also include lower urinary tract signs and symptoms.[4] Laboratory criteria are the same as for AUC.[4]

UTI involving the bladder and/or kidneys is generally classified as complicated or uncomplicated. Complicated UTI is defined as an infection occurring in a patient with comorbid medical conditions and/or anatomic abnormalities of the urinary tract that may increase the difficulty of diagnosing UTI as well as the likelihood of various adverse outcomes, such as a resistant causative bacteria, delayed or inadequate response to antimicrobial therapy, a need for prolonged therapy or hospitalization, and significant morbidity.[5] Commonly encountered complicating factors for UTI include pregnancy, functional bladder abnormalities such as neurogenic bladder, renal transplant, urinary stones, structural abnormalities of the urinary tract, diabetes, male gender, urinary catheterization or instrumentation, recent hospitalization or antibiotic exposure, and advanced age. Most complicating factors are also important host factors in the pathogenesis of UTI.

PATHOPHYSIOLOGY
Overview of UTI Pathogenesis: Bacterial Uropathogenesis and Interplay with Host Factors

Although this article focuses on host factors in the pathogenesis of UTI, a brief review of bacterial factors in UTI is relevant, given the interplay of host susceptibility and bacterial virulence that occurs in most infections. UTI has served as an excellent model of bacterial pathogenesis throughout years of study in multiple laboratories, with most studies focusing on virulence traits of *Escherichia coli*, the most common cause of UTI in all age groups and clinical settings.[6] Although the busy clinician is appropriately currently focused on diagnosis, treatment, and prevention of UTI, some of the genetic susceptibility issues discussed here relate to specific host responses to bacterial traits. At least for children, there is a possibility in the near future of using genetic testing to detect specific genetically determined susceptibility to pyelonephritis.[6] In addition, some newer preventive measures, discussed in the article by Geerlings and colleagues elsewhere in this issue, are based on specific findings learned through detailed study of bacterial pathogenesis in UTI.

As noted, *E coli* causes 80% to 90% of AUC or AUP in young, healthy, sexually active women,[7] as well as most complicated UTIs.[8] *E coli* are generally divided into intestinal pathogens and extraintestinal *E coli* (ExPEC), based on the disease syndromes linked to the organisms epidemiologically. Numerous laboratory-based and clinical-epidemiologic studies have demonstrated a subset of ExPEC specifically associated with UTI, the uropathogenic *E coli* (UPEC), organisms expressing traits rendering them specially adapted to express virulence and fitness in the urinary tract of humans and animal models.[9] The specific adaptations of UPEC include virulence determinants and fitness factors that allow the bacteria to successfully subvert or hijack host defenses so as to initially attach to urogenital mucosal surfaces, to then interact with these tissues by setting off cascades of signaling and other immunologic response events, and even to invade the bladder. These UPEC adaptations include fimbrial and nonfimbrial adhesins for initial attachment to the mucosa; metal acquisition systems for living in environments such as urine that are poor in iron and other needed metals; toxins for breaching barriers, destroying host defense cells, and releasing needed nutrient molecules; flagellae for swimming motion; inactivators of host defenses such as enterobactin; and fimbrial phase variation mechanisms that can change the antigens seen by the host faster than the host can adapt.[10] Through these manifold adaptations to the urinary tract, UPEC has proven itself a formidable opponent, capable of survival and rapid adaptation in the relatively hostile environment of urine. Although clinically relevant primarily in outbreak investigations, UPEC can be identified serologically or genetically by typing methods that detect surface antigens (OKH) or specific virulence determinants.[6] Furthermore, certain UPEC virulence determinants are being investigated as possible UTI vaccine targets,[11] as described in greater detail in the article by Geerlings and colleagues, elsewhere in this issue.

HOST FACTORS IN UTI

From a clinical standpoint, understanding the pathogenesis of UTI is helpful in predicting and attempting to prevent recurrences, and for patient education. Accordingly, host factors relevant to UTI are presented here as either potentially modifiable factors or factors that cannot likely be modified, but are important to understanding the likelihood of UTI, especially recurrent infections, and may be areas of intervention in the future.

Potentially Modifiable Host Factors in UTI

Behavioral factors

Key behavioral risk factors for AUC and AUP in women, including both recurrent and sporadic AUC, are sexual intercourse, the use of spermicides for contraception, and a new sexual partner within the past year.[12,13] Clinical studies of women before and immediately following sexual intercourse indicate that intercourse increases the risk of bacteriuria for at least 24 hours afterward, especially in women using spermicides for contraception.[12] Likewise, frequency of recent sexual intercourse is correlated with the rate of UTI.[7] Some women notice a temporal association of recurrent UTI with intercourse, and thus may benefit from consideration of a postcoital prophylactic regimen (discussed in greater detail elsewhere in this issue).[14] Although data supporting the efficacy of voiding before and/or after intercourse are scant,[4] this measure is commonly adopted by women suffering from frequent recurrences. Other behaviors that may seem logically related to the risk of UTI, such as wiping habits or hydration status, have not been shown to be associative, but it is not known whether this is because most women studied had already modified these behaviors.[4]

Antimicrobial exposure

Some years ago, antecedent antimicrobial exposure was shown to increase the subsequent relative risk of UTI in healthy premenopausal women, whether the antimicrobial therapy was given for treatment of UTI or for other infections.[15] The pathogenesis of this effect was postulated to be alterations in the normal microbiota of the urogenital mucosae, especially the vaginal microbiota, which normally contains protective lactobacilli.[15] Increasing evidence indicates that antimicrobial exposure is also associated with subsequent, relatively durable resistance to commonly used antimicrobials for UTI. In a recent study comparing cranberry capsules with antimicrobials (trimethoprim/sulfamethoxazole [TMP/SMX]), subjects receiving the active antimicrobial therapy had a significantly increased risk of resistance to TMP/SMX among fecal and asymptomatic bacteriuria (ASB) isolates collected 1 month after therapy, compared with subjects receiving cranberry.[16] A systematic review and meta-analysis of antimicrobial prescribing in primary care showed that patients receiving antimicrobials for a respiratory infection or UTI developed resistance to the agent prescribed, with the greatest effect observed in the first month after treatment, but persisting up to 12 months in some cases.[17] A study of pediatric outpatients with their first diagnosis of UTI found that recent antimicrobial exposure was associated with antimicrobial-resistant UTIs in this population.[18] The clinical implications from these and many corroborative studies are that whenever feasible, antimicrobial sparing may reduce the risk of UTI and of acquisition of resistant bacteria in individual patients. This information may also be useful in patient education regarding UTIs.

Urogenital microbiota

The urogenital and intestinal microbiota plays important roles in the pathogenesis of UTI, particularly in women. The ultimate source of uropathogenic E coli and other uropathogens is the intestinal tract, as demonstrated in numerous studies.[19–21] In women, especially for E coli, colonization of the vaginal introitus and urethra with organisms from the rectal microbiota is the critical event preceding UTI.[19–21] In addition, among women with frequently recurrent UTI, vaginal colonization with E coli or other Enterobacteriaceae is more common, prolonged, and persistent than in women who do not develop a pattern of recurrences.[22–24]

The increased vaginal and periurethral colonization with enteric organisms seen just before UTI (and at baseline in women with recurrent UTI) is accompanied by a concomitant loss of the normally predominant and protective vaginal lactobacilli.[22–24] Both culture-based and genomics-based studies demonstrate the prevalence of Lactobacillus spp in the vaginal microbiota.[25–28] In clinical studies, women lacking vaginal lactobacilli, particularly H_2O_2-producing lactobacilli, are at increased risk for bacterial vaginosis, human immunodeficiency virus, and Neisseria gonorrhoeae, as well as vaginal colonization with E coli.[29–34] Proposed mechanisms through which lactobacilli may prevent vaginal colonization by uropathogens include competitive exclusion of E coli by adherence of Lactobacillus spp to uroepithelial cells; lowering of vaginal pH by production of lactic acid; production of bacteriocins, surfactants, and other antimicrobial products; and production of H_2O_2.[35–42] Hydrogen peroxide alone is microbicidal for many bacterial species, and this microbicidal activity is 10- to 100-fold greater when it is combined with chloride anion and myeloperoxidase, both of which are found in the vagina.[19,43] This vaginal antimicrobial defense system (H_2O_2, chloride anion, and myeloperoxidase) has potent in vitro activity against E coli and other microorganisms.[44]

Several exposures are associated with the loss of normally prevalent and protective lactobacilli and with an increased risk of UTI, including exposure to spermicides[12,24,45] or β-lactam antimicrobials, which may simply kill the lactobacilli. These differential collateral effects of β-lactam agents, disrupting the protective vaginal microbiota more than agents such as TMP/SMX and often proving less efficacious than agents without these effects in clinical trials, are reflected in current guidelines for management of AUC and AUP published by the Infectious Diseases Society of America.[46–48] A physiologic condition associated with a decrease in or total loss of lactobacilli, an elevated vaginal pH, and increased risk of UTI is the normal loss of estrogen at the menopause, surgical or natural.[49] In bacterial vaginosis, lactobacilli are depleted, and the dysbiosis that results may include increased colonization with *E coli* and association with UTI in some studies.[23]

As discussed in greater detail in the article by Geerlings and colleagues elsewhere in this issue, a new method of preventing recurrent UTI is the use of *Lactobacillus* probiotic preparations given vaginally.[50] A recent small random-effects model meta-analysis, when data were subjected to a sensitivity analysis excluding studies using ineffective strains and studies testing for safety, showed that among 127 patients in 2 studies, a statistically significant decrease in recurrent UTI was found in patients given a *Lactobacillus* probiotic, denoted by the pooled risk ratio of 0.51 (95% confidence interval 0.26–0.99; $P = .05$) with no statistical heterogeneity ($I^2 = 0$%).[50] The investigators concluded that although probiotic strains of *Lactobacillus* seem safe and effective in preventing recurrent UTI in adult women, larger randomized clinical trials (RCTs) are required before definitive recommendations may be made.[50] In the United States, RCTs of promising probiotic products for the prevention of UTI are ongoing.

Fecal microbiota and bladder invasion

The fecal microbiota also plays a role in the pathogenesis of UTI, serving as a reservoir for infection and recurrences. As in sporadic UTI, UPEC is the most common cause of recurrent AUC.[51] Clinical and molecular epidemiologic studies of recurrent UPEC UTI in women have shown that the overwhelming majority of these episodes are reinfections, usually with the same strain of UPEC that often persists in the fecal microbiota for 12 months or more, repeatedly circulating through the fecal and vaginal reservoirs to cause recurrences of AUC.[52–54] Some studies of probiotics to prevent recurrent UTI have used oral preparations,[55] although detailed studies of the distal intestinal microbiome in UTI and the effects of probiotics in these microbiota are not yet available.

In addition to the fecal reservoir in the pathogenesis of UTI, elegant mouse models of UTI have demonstrated that UPEC invade the bladder epithelium and form intracellular bacterial communities (IBC) and quiescent intracellular reservoirs, complex intracellular systems associated with resistance to clearance by antimicrobial treatment and recrudescence of bacteriuria.[56] Although a detailed prospective cohort study of microbiological and inflammatory events in the 2 weeks preceding UPEC recurrent UTI in women supported an ascending model of UTI with a fecal-vaginal reservoir in virtually all patients studied,[52] IBC-like structures have been identified in exfoliated uroepithelial cells collected from women with AUC.[57] Thus, although fecal and vaginal reservoirs of UPEC are clearly critical in UTI pathogenesis, evidence supports intracellular sequestration of UPEC within the human bladder. Clinically and molecularly, this phenomenon is an active area of UTI research that, it is hoped, will yield clinical answers regarding especially recalcitrant recurrent infections.

Lack of estrogen post menopause

As already described, the loss of estrogen at the menopause is known to result in a decrement or complete loss in vaginal lactobacilli.[49] However, a recent study of estrogen effects using clinical samples from a small number of premenopausal and postmenopausal women, as well as animal and in vitro human urothelial cell models, indicated that other key urogenital mucosal host defense mechanisms are also associated with estrogen.[58] Investigating serum levels of one antimicrobial peptide, a key element of innate immunity, and exfoliated urothelial expression levels of 5 other antimicrobial peptides, the group found differential effects among samples collected from premenopausal and postmenopausal women, with most peptides lower in samples from postmenopausal women.[58] These antimicrobial peptide expression levels increased with estrogen supplementation.[58] In addition, most samples from the post-menopausal women studied showed greater urothelial cell shedding during UTI, indicating possible compromise of epithelial barrier functions.[58] Accordingly, some key epithelial barrier function proteins were reduced in samples from postmenopausal women, and upregulated with estrogen supplementation.[58] The key findings were reproduced in experiments with a mouse model and urothelial cell lines.[58] In summary, estrogen seems to promote not only a protective vaginal microbiota but also a protective bladder epithelium, with more robust barrier functions and higher production of antimicrobial peptides.[58]

Anatomic and functional problems of the urinary tract

Although details of UTI among patients with anatomic and functional abnormalities of the urinary tract is included in the section on complicated UTIs, it is important to remember that these comorbid conditions defining complicated UTI also highlight key mechanical and functional host factors in the pathogenesis of UTI. For example, an obstructed urinary tract predisposes to infection, and when obstructed pyelonephritis occurs it is considered a urologic emergency requiring immediate decompression.[59] Infected renal calculi may also be associated with severe morbidity, such as sepsis.[60] A prospective cohort study of hospitalized patients found that bacteremia secondary to *E coli* bacteriuria was frequent (15%) in patients who were tested for it.[61] Symptoms of urinary obstruction independently predicted bacteremia, as did procedures that involved surgical breach of urogenital tissues.[61] Clinically, any reversible anatomic or functional abnormalities of the urinary tract should be promptly addressed as much as is feasible.

Nonmodifiable Host Factors in UTI

Female gender

Except in the first year of life, females are disproportionately affected by UTI.[62] Approximately one-half to one-third of women self-report having had at least 1 episode of UTI requiring treatment by the age of 32 years.[62] A prospective study of AUC among sexually active women aged 18 to 40 years without a history of recurrent UTI attending a university clinic or a health maintenance organization (HMO) in Seattle demonstrated an incidence of AUC of 0.5 to 0.7 per person-year.[7] A population-based, prospective cohort study of postmenopausal women aged 55 to 75 years receiving care in the same HMO showed an incidence of AUC of 0.07 per person-year.[63]

Although gender is usually a nonmodifiable risk factor, the predilection of women for developing UTI can be used as a starting point for patient discussions of the pathogenesis of UTI, clinically relevant risk factors, and measures patients can take to reduce risk.

Genetics as a host factor in UTI

Epidemiologic data Several epidemiologic studies provide evidence of inherited host factors predisposing to UTI. It has long been known that a personal history of prior UTI is a risk factor for recurrent infection, as shown in a seminal longitudinal study of patients attending a clinic for recurrent and complicated UTI.[64] Subsequently, findings in a large case-control study of healthy premenopausal women with and without a history of recurrent UTI showing that a history of first UTI before age 15 and a maternal history of UTI were associated with an increased risk of recurrent UTI suggested a genetic component.[13] These data were corroborated in 2 subsequent epidemiologic studies. A population-based case-control study of AUP among women receiving care in a prepaid health plan showed that patient and family history of UTI are associated with an increased risk of AUP.[65] In a population-based case-control study of

1261 women 18 to 49 years old enrolled in a prepaid health plan, a history of UTI in female relatives was strongly and consistently associated with recurrent AUC and AUP.[66] The risk increased with the number of affected relatives, reinforcing the concept of a genetic influence on susceptibility to UTI.[66]

Innate immune associations To further elucidate the possible roles of heritable factors in the pathogenesis of UTI, most studies have focused on innate immune defenses. The innate immune system is critical to the host response to UTI, as shown in animal models and in studies of children with innate immune defects predisposing them to UTI, especially AUP.[6] As in any mucosal infection, toll-like receptors (TLR) are key initial molecules in the pathogenic cascade of UTI.[6] Bacterial recognition of TLR leads to cytokine and chemokine responses and recruitment of inflammatory cells; TLR1 and TLR2, recognizing lipopeptide, TLR4, recognizing lipopolysaccharide, and TLR5, recognizing flagellin, are particularly relevant to *E coli* uropathogenesis. Various effector molecules are activated through interaction with TLRs, including chemokines and transcription factors such as IRF3. In studies of single-nucleotide polymorphisms (SNPs) in TLR pathways and effector molecules, various SNPs in TLR pathway genes have been associated with a reduction or increase in risk of UTI or ASB.[6,67–69]

Among children and in animal models, mutations that reduce TLR4 expression or function are associated with ASB, and SNPs that reduce the effector molecule IRF3 or the expression of the chemokine CXCR1 are associated with AUP and an increased risk of renal scarring.[6,69] In a population-based case-control study of SNPs in 9 TLR pathway genes among women aged 18 to 49 years, including 431 recurrent UTI cases, 400 AUP cases, and 430 controls with no history of UTIs, an SNP in TLR4 was associated with protection from recurrent UTI but not pyelonephritis, whereas an SNP in TLR5 that abrogates flagellin-induced signaling was associated with an increased risk of recurrent UTI but not AUP.[67] An SNP in TLR1 was associated with protection from AUP.[67] These associations were modest, but in studies in of ASB in 1261 asymptomatic women aged 18 to 49 years, an SNP in TLR2 was associated with associated with increased risk of ASB (odds ratio 3.44).[68] Because ASB often precedes the development of acute UTI,[70] taken together the findings from these studies suggest that at least in adult females, genetic factors such as innate immune response variants affect in vivo host responses from the point of introduction of bacteria into the bladder.[68]

At present, studies of innate immune response variations are restricted to the realm of research. However, in children the ability to predict a risk of recurrent UTI has been proposed as having potential future utility in decision making regarding invasive surgical procedures to correct anatomic anomalies.[6] Another possible application might be in renal transplantation, for which studies of early expression of innate immune responses are beginning to distinguish predictors of allograft status.[71]

SUMMARY AND DISCUSSION

UTIs are among the most common infections encountered in clinical care of both outpatients and hospitalized patients throughout the life span. Girls and women are disproportionately affected except in the first year of life. Annual rates of ambulatory visits in the United States for UTI likely exceed the 8.6 million ambulatory visits by both men and women when last quantified in 2007 through the CDC NHAMCS. Clinically, host factors in the pathogenesis of UTI may be considered as modifiable and, thus, potentially amenable to a change in patient behavior or treatment approach, or as intrinsic and nonmodifiable host factors that neither the patient nor the clinician can influence. Examples of potentially modifiable factors include behaviors associated with an increased risk of UTI, such as sexual intercourse or choice of contraceptive; recent exposure to antimicrobials; characteristics of the urogenital or fecal microbiota; some anatomic and functional problems of the urinary tract that may be treatable; and lack of estrogen stemming from surgical or natural menopause. Patients may be able to change contraceptive methods, and clinicians can spare antimicrobial therapy to only clearly necessary treatments, given the risks of both UTI and multidrug-resistant bacteria that are associated with antimicrobial therapy. Therapeutic interventions to address alterations in the urogenital microbiota are currently being studied, and estrogen therapy may help some postmenopausal women with frequently recurrent UTIs.

Intrinsic, nonmodifiable host factors in UTI include gender and genetic influences, largely differences in innate immune host functions associated with the pathogenesis of UTI. Although considering nonmodifiable host factors may be discouraging to patients and clinicians at present, some genetic associations have the potential for future predictive value and may interface with future treatments.

REFERENCES

1. Schappert SM, Rechtsteiner EA. Ambulatory medical care utilization estimates for 2007. Vital Health Stat 13 2011;(169):1–38.
2. Foxman B, Brown P. Epidemiology of urinary tract infections: transmission and risk factors, incidence, and costs. Infect Dis Clin North Am 2003;17(2): 227–41.
3. Hooton T. The current management strategies for community-acquired urinary tract infection. Infect Dis Clin North Am 2003;17:303–32.
4. Hooton TM. Clinical practice. Uncomplicated urinary tract infection. N Engl J Med 2012;366(11):1028–37.
5. Nicolle LE. Complicated urinary tract infection in adults. Can J Infect Dis Med Microbiol 2005;16(6):349–60.
6. Ragnarsdottir B, Svanborg C. Susceptibility to acute pyelonephritis or asymptomatic bacteriuria: host-pathogen interaction in urinary tract infections. Pediatr Nephrol 2012;27(11):2017–29.
7. Hooton TM, Scholes D, Hughes JP, et al. A prospective study of risk factors for symptomatic urinary tract infection in young women. N Engl J Med 1996;335(7): 468–74.
8. Johnson J. Microbial virulence determinants and the pathogenesis of urinary tract infection. Infect Dis Clin North Am 2003;17:261–78, viii.
9. Stapleton AE. Urinary tract infection in women: new pathogenic considerations. Curr Infect Dis Rep 2006;8(6):465–72.
10. Nielubowicz GR, Mobley HL. Host-pathogen interactions in urinary tract infection. Nat Rev Urol 2010;7(8):430–41.
11. Brumbaugh AR, Mobley HL. Preventing urinary tract infection: progress toward an effective Escherichia coli vaccine. Expert Rev Vaccines 2012;11(6): 663–76.
12. Hooton TM, Hillier S, Johnson C, et al. Escherichia coli bacteriuria and contraceptive method. JAMA 1991;265(1):64–9.
13. Scholes D, Hooton TM, Roberts PL, et al. Risk factors for recurrent urinary tract infection in young women. J Infect Dis 2000;182(4):1177–82.
14. Stapleton A, Latham RH, Johnson C, et al. Postcoital antimicrobial prophylaxis for recurrent urinary tract infection. A randomized, double-blind, placebo-controlled trial. JAMA 1990;264(6):703–6.

15. Smith HS, Hughes JP, Hooton TM, et al. Antecedent antimicrobial use increases the risk of uncomplicated cystitis in young women. Clin Infect Dis 1997;25(1):63–8.
16. Beerepoot MJ, ter Riet G, Nys S, et al. Cranberries vs antibiotics to prevent urinary tract infections: a randomized double-blind noninferiority trial in premenopausal women. Arch Intern Med 2011;171(14):1270–8.
17. Costelloe C, Metcalfe C, Lovering A, et al. Effect of antibiotic prescribing in primary care on antimicrobial resistance in individual patients: systematic review and meta-analysis. BMJ 2010;340:c2096.
18. Paschke AA, Zaoutis T, Conway PH, et al. Previous antimicrobial exposure is associated with drug-resistant urinary tract infections in children. Pediatrics 2010;125(4):664–72.
19. Hooton TM, Stamm WE. The vaginal flora and urinary tract infections. In: Warren JW, Mobley HL, editors. Urinary tract infections: molecular pathogenesis and clinical management. Washington, DC: ASM Press; 1996. p. 67.
20. Pfau A, Sacks T. The bacterial flora of the vaginal vestibule, urethra and vagina in premenopausal women with recurrent urinary tract infections. J Urol 1981;126(5):630–4.
21. Stamey TA, Sexton CC. The role of vaginal colonization with Enterobacteriaceae in recurrent urinary tract infections. J Urol 1975;113:214–7.
22. Gupta K, Stapleton AE, Hooton TM, et al. Inverse association of H_2O_2-producing lactobacilli and vaginal *Escherichia coli* colonization in women with recurrent urinary tract infections. J Infect Dis 1998;178(2):446–50.
23. Hooton TM, Fihn SD, Johnson C, et al. Association between bacterial vaginosis and acute cystitis in women using diaphragms. Arch Intern Med 1989;149(9):1932–6.
24. Hooton TM, Roberts PL, Stamm WE. Effects of recent sexual activity and use of a diaphragm on the vaginal microflora. Clin Infect Dis 1994;19(2):274–8.
25. Antonio MA, Hawes SE, Hillier SL. The identification of vaginal *Lactobacillus* species and the demographic and microbiologic characteristics of women colonized by these species. J Infect Dis 1999;180(6):1950–6.
26. Ravel J, Gajer P, Abdo Z, et al. Vaginal microbiome of reproductive-age women. Proc Natl Acad Sci U S A 2011;108(Suppl 1):4680–7.
27. Zhou X, Brown CJ, Abdo Z, et al. Differences in the composition of vaginal microbial communities found in healthy Caucasian and black women. ISME J 2007;1(2):121–33.
28. Zhou X, Hansmann MA, Davis CC, et al. The vaginal bacterial communities of Japanese women resemble those of women in other racial groups. FEMS Immunol Med Microbiol 2010;58(2):169–81.
29. Hawes SE, Hillier SL, Benedetti J, et al. Hydrogen peroxide-producing lactobacilli and acquisition of vaginal infections. J Infect Dis 1996;174:1058–63.
30. Martin HL, Richardson BA, Nyange PM, et al. Vaginal lactobacilli, microbial flora, and risk of human immunodeficiency virus type 1 and sexually transmitted disease acquisition. J Infect Dis 1999;180(6):1863–8.
31. Schwebke JR. Role of vaginal flora as a barrier to HIV acquisition. Curr Infect Dis Rep 2001;3(2):152–5.
32. Taha TE, Hoover DR, Dallabetta GA, et al. Bacterial vaginosis and disturbances of vaginal flora: association with increased acquisition of HIV. AIDS 1998;12(13):1699–706.
33. van De Wijgert JH, Mason PR, Gwanzura L, et al. Intravaginal practices, vaginal flora disturbances, and acquisition of sexually transmitted diseases in Zimbabwean women. J Infect Dis 2000;181(2):587–94.

34. Zheng HY, Alcorn TM, Cohen MS. Effects of H_2O_2-producing lactobacilli on *Neisseria gonorrhoeae* growth and catalase activity. J Infect Dis 1994;170(5): 1209–15.
35. Boris S, Barbes C. Role played by lactobacilli in controlling the population of vaginal pathogens. Microbes Infect 2000;2(5):543–6.
36. Herthelius M, Gorbach SL, Mollby R, et al. Elimination of vaginal colonization with *Escherichia coli* by administration of indigenous flora. Infect Immun 1989; 57(8):2447–51.
37. McGroarty JA, Reid G. Detection of a *Lactobacillus* substance that inhibits *Escherichia coli*. Can J Microbiol 1988;34(8):974–8.
38. McGroarty JA, Tomeczek L, Pond DG, et al. Hydrogen peroxide production by *Lactobacillus* species: correlation with susceptibility to the spermicidal compound nonoxynol-9. J Infect Dis 1992;165(6):1142–4.
39. Osset J, Bartolome RM, Garcia E, et al. Assessment of the capacity of *Lactobacillus* to inhibit the growth of uropathogens and block their adhesion to vaginal epithelial cells. J Infect Dis 2001;183(3):485–91.
40. Reid G, Cook RL, Bruce AW. Examination of strains of lactobacilli for properties that may influence bacterial interference in the urinary tract. J Urol 1987;138(2): 330–5.
41. Reid G, Heinemann C, Velraeds M, et al. Biosurfactants produced by *Lactobacillus*. Meth Enzymol 1999;310:426–33.
42. Stamey TA, Kaufman MF. Studies of introital colonization in women with recurrent urinary infections. II. A comparison of growth in normal vaginal fluid of common versus uncommon serogroups of *Escherichia coli*. J Urol 1975; 114(2):264–7.
43. Schaeffer AJ, Jones JM, Amundsen SK. Bacterial effect of hydrogen peroxide on urinary tract pathogens. Appl Environ Microbiol 1980;40(2):337–40.
44. Klebanoff SJ, Hillier SL, Eschenbach DA, et al. Control of the microbial flora of the vagina by H_2O_2-generating lactobacilli. J Infect Dis 1991;164:94–100.
45. Hooton TM, Fennell CL, Clark AM, et al. Nonoxynol-9: differential antibacterial activity and enhancement of bacterial adherence to vaginal epithelial cells. J Infect Dis 1991;164(6):1216–9.
46. Hooton TM, Scholes D, Gupta K, et al. Amoxicillin-clavulanate vs ciprofloxacin for the treatment of uncomplicated cystitis in women: a randomized trial. JAMA 2005;293(8):949–55.
47. Hooton TM, Roberts PL, Stapleton AE. Cefpodoxime vs ciprofloxacin for short-course treatment of acute uncomplicated cystitis: a randomized trial. JAMA 2012;307(6):583–9.
48. Gupta K, Hooton TM, Naber KG, et al. International clinical practice guidelines for the treatment of acute uncomplicated cystitis and pyelonephritis in women: a 2010 update by the Infectious Diseases Society of America and the European Society for Microbiology and Infectious Diseases. Clin Infect Dis 2011;52(5): e103–20.
49. Raz R. Urinary tract infection in postmenopausal women. Korean J Urol 2011; 52(12):801–8.
50. Grin PM, Kowalewska PM, Alhazzan W, et al. *Lactobacillus* for preventing recurrent urinary tract infections in women: meta-analysis. Can J Urol 2013;20(1): 6607–14.
51. Stapleton A, Moseley S, Stamm WE. Urovirulence determinants in *Escherichia coli* isolates causing first-episode and recurrent cystitis in women. J Infect Dis 1991;163(4):773–9.

52. Czaja CA, Stamm WE, Stapleton AE, et al. Prospective cohort study of microbial and inflammatory events immediately preceding *Escherichia coli* recurrent urinary tract infection in women. J Infect Dis 2009;200(4):528–36.
53. Hooton TM. Recurrent urinary tract infection in women. Int J Antimicrob Agents 2001;17(4):259–68.
54. Russo TA, Stapleton A, Wenderoth S, et al. Chromosomal restriction fragment length polymorphism analysis of *Escherichia coli* strains causing recurrent urinary tract infections in young women. J Infect Dis 1995;172(2):440–5.
55. Beerepoot MA, ter Riet G, Nys S, et al. Lactobacilli vs antibiotics to prevent urinary tract infections: a randomized, double-blind, noninferiority trial in post-menopausal women. Arch Intern Med 2012;172(9):704–12.
56. Hannan TJ, Totsika M, Mansfield KJ, et al. Host-pathogen checkpoints and population bottlenecks in persistent and intracellular uropathogenic *Escherichia coli* bladder infection. FEMS Microbiol Rev 2012;36(3):616–48.
57. Rosen DA, Hooton TM, Stamm WE, et al. Detection of intracellular bacterial communities in human urinary tract infection. PLoS Med 2007;4(12):e329.
58. Luthje P, Brauner H, Ramos NL, et al. Estrogen supports urothelial defense mechanisms. Sci Transl Med 2013;5(190):190ra180.
59. Matlaga BR. How do we manage infected, obstructed hydronephrosis? Eur Urol 2013;64(1):93–4.
60. Sammon JD, Ghani KR, Karakiewicz PI, et al. Temporal trends, practice patterns, and treatment outcomes for infected upper urinary tract stones in the United States. Eur Urol 2013;64(1):85–92.
61. Marschall J, Zhang L, Foxman B, et al. Both host and pathogen factors predispose to *Escherichia coli* urinary-source bacteremia in hospitalized patients. Clin Infect Dis 2012;54(12):1692–8.
62. Foxman B. Epidemiology of urinary tract infections: incidence, morbidity, and economic costs. Dis Mon 2003;49(2):53–70.
63. Jackson SL, Boyko EJ, Scholes D, et al. Predictors of urinary tract infection after menopause: a prospective study. Am J Med 2004;117(12):903–11.
64. Stamm WE, McKevitt M, Roberts PL, et al. Natural history of recurrent urinary tract infections in women. Rev Infect Dis 1991;13:77–84.
65. Scholes D, Hooton TM, Roberts PL, et al. Risk factors associated with acute pyelonephritis in healthy women. Ann Intern Med 2005;142(1):20–7.
66. Scholes D, Hawn TR, Roberts PL, et al. Family history and risk of recurrent cystitis and pyelonephritis in women. J Urol 2010;184(2):564–9.
67. Hawn TR, Scholes D, Li SS, et al. Toll-like receptor polymorphisms and susceptibility to urinary tract infections in adult women. PLoS One 2009;4(6):e5990.
68. Hawn TR, Scholes D, Wang H, et al. Genetic variation of the human urinary tract innate immune response and asymptomatic bacteriuria in women. PLoS One 2009;4(12):e8300.
69. Ragnarsdottir B, Samuelsson M, Gustafsson MC, et al. Reduced toll-like receptor 4 expression in children with asymptomatic bacteriuria. J Infect Dis 2007; 196(3):475–84.
70. Hooton TM, Scholes D, Stapleton AE, et al. A prospective study of asymptomatic bacteriuria in sexually active young women [see comments]. N Engl J Med 2000;343(14):992–7.
71. McDaniel DO, Rigney DA, McDaniel KY, et al. Early expression profile of inflammatory markers and kidney allograft status. Transplant Proc 2013;45(4):1523.

Index

Note: Page numbers of article titles are in **boldface** type.

Infect Dis Clin N Am 28 (2014) 161–167
http://dx.doi.org/10.1016/S0891-5520(13)00112-8
0891-5520/14/$ – see front matter © 2014 Elsevier Inc. All rights reserved.

id.theclinics.com

Moving?

Make sure your subscription moves with you!

To notify us of your new address, find your **Clinics Account Number** (located on your mailing label above your name), and contact customer service at:

Email: journalscustomerservice-usa@elsevier.com

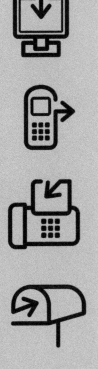

800-654-2452 (subscribers in the U.S. & Canada)
314-447-8871 (subscribers outside of the U.S. & Canada)

Fax number: 314-447-8029

Elsevier Health Sciences Division
Subscription Customer Service
3251 Riverport Lane
Maryland Heights, MO 63043

*To ensure uninterrupted delivery of your subscription, please notify us at least 4 weeks in advance of move.

Printed and bound by CPI Group (UK) Ltd, Croydon, CR0 4YY

07/10/2024

01040498-0017